Implementing the Expressive Therapies Continuum

Implementing the Expressive Therapies Continuum aims to explore the use of the Expressive Therapies Continuum (ETC) in the form of specific expressive therapy initiatives intended to be used in both educational and professional settings. Drawing on materials codeveloped by Dr. Sandra Graves-Alcorn, coauthor and developer of the ETC, as well as tried and tested curriculum by Professor Christa Kagin, this interdisciplinary resource will be of great value to students, teachers, and mental health clinicians, as well as other health-care practitioners interested in utilizing the ETC developmental model. All of this is delivered in a clear and easy-to-follow presentation designed to engage readers.

Sandra Graves-Alcorn, PhD, was one of the charter members of the American Art Therapy Association and has served as its chair of education, standards chair, peer review chair, president-elect and president. She developed the master's degree in art therapy at the University of Louisville in 1969 and went on to found the Institute of Expressive Therapies, which she chaired for several years. She was also chair of the Department of Art Therapy when it transferred to Allied Health in the School of Medicine. Sandra is the author of *Expressions of Healing: Embracing the Process of Grief*, published by Newcastle in 1994. She has also authored numerous articles and has made professional presentations throughout the United States and Canada. She also co-owned and operated a national bereavement service company and was president and owner of two counseling agencies as well as a foster care provider. She has received many awards and was granted Outstanding Alumni at the University of Louisville.

Sandra now resides in Florida with her husband Wayne. She may be contacted by email at sandragravesalcorn@gmail.com.

Christa Kagin, MA-ATR, is chair of the Art Department at Benedictine College in Atchison, Kansas, where she teaches painting, art history, and art therapy courses (for an undergraduate specialization in art therapy). She has been past president of the Kansas Art Therapy Association and is still an active member. When she is not teaching or providing art therapy services through private practice and community service, she is a mom to three wonderful children and wife to a wonderful man.

She resides in rural Kansas, where her view of the stars is spectacular!

"This book describes an extensive array of activities to be used with students or clients, depending on the art therapist's goals. Based on the Expressive Therapies Continuum and Media Dimension Variables, the exercises are presented clearly and explicitly, enabling the teacher or therapist to easily present them to those they serve. Along with the specific directives are explanations of the theories on which they are based, a useful addition to anyone's clinical or educational armamentarium."

Judith A. Rubin, *PhD, ATR-BC, HLM, president,*
Expressive Media, Inc.

"This volume expands clinical applications of the Expressive Therapies Continuum in a way that no other book has to date. The authors have articulated a rich variety of art-based processes through a series of pragmatic, user-friendly examples and brain-wise concepts. This book will introduce helping professionals to new ways of approaching their work and inspire practitioners in the fields of creative arts therapies, counseling, psychology, and education to expand their repertoire of creative interventions with children, adults, families and groups."

Cathy Malchiodi, *PhD, LPCC, LPAT, ATR-BC, REAT,*
executive director, Trauma-Informed Practices and
Expressive Arts Therapy Institute, Louisville, Kentucky

"This personal, intimate, and highly readable book will be useful to both beginning and experienced art therapists, as well as those in movement/dance, music, drama and poetry therapy. One of the book's compelling strengths is its comfortable, user-friendly writing style, infused throughout with an intimate tone. With easy to follow suggestions, they lead one on to ever widening explorations toward greater self-awareness."

Eleanor Irwin, *PhD, drama therapist, RDT, clinical*
assistant professor of psychiatry, University of Pittsburgh

"Graves and Kagin have provided clinicians with a carefully sequenced, powerful, and elegant method that will deepen clients' expressive capacities and personal exploration. The Expressive Therapies Continuum remains one of the most important systemic approaches in our field, and this book benefits from the authors' years of experience in a wide range of settings. I highly recommend this to all expressive arts therapists, clinicians, and teachers interested in the potential of the creative act to heal."

David Read Johnson, *PhD, RDT-BCT, co-director, Post Traumatic*
Stress Center, New Haven, Connecticut, associate clinical professor in
the Department of Psychiatry, Yale University School of Medicine

Implementing the Expressive Therapies Continuum

A Guide for Clinical Practice

Sandra Graves-Alcorn
and Christa Kagin

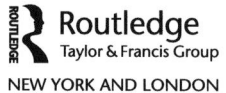

Routledge
Taylor & Francis Group
NEW YORK AND LONDON

First published 2017
by Routledge
711 Third Avenue, New York, NY 10017

and by Routledge
2 Park Square, Milton Park, Abingdon, Oxon, OX14 4RN

Routledge is an imprint of the Taylor & Francis Group, an informa business

© 2017 Taylor & Francis

The right of Sandra Graves-Alcorn and Christa Kagin to be identified as authors of this work has been asserted by them in accordance with sections 77 and 78 of the Copyright, Designs and Patents Act 1988.

All rights reserved. No part of this book may be reprinted or reproduced or utilised in any form or by any electronic, mechanical, or other means, now known or hereafter invented, including photocopying and recording, or in any information storage or retrieval system, without permission in writing from the publishers.

Trademark notice: Product or corporate names may be trademarks or registered trademarks, and are used only for identification and explanation without intent to infringe.

Library of Congress Cataloging-in-Publication Data
Names: Graves-Alcorn, Sandra, author. | Kagin, Christa, author.
Title: Implementing the expressive therapies continuum : a guide for clinical practice / Sandra Graves-Alcorn and Christa Kagin.
Description: New York : Routledge, 2017. | Includes bibliographical references and index.
Identifiers: LCCN 2016043515 | ISBN 9781138652385 (hbk. : alk. paper) | ISBN 9781138652408 (pbk. : alk. paper) | ISBN 9781315624303 (e-book)
Subjects: MESH: Art Therapy—methods | Creativity
Classification: LCC RC489.A7 | NLM WM 450.5.A8 | DDC 616.89/1656—dc23
LC record available at https://lccn.loc.gov/2016043515

ISBN: 978-1-138-65238-5 (hbk)
ISBN: 978-1-138-65240-8 (pbk)
ISBN: 978-1-315-62430-3 (ebk)

Typeset in ITC Giovanni Std
by Apex CoVantage, LLC

[T]he existence of human beings will never be satisfactorily explained in terms of isolated instincts or purposive mechanism such as hunger, power, sex, survival, perpetuation of the species. [T]hat is man's main purpose is not to eat, drink, etc. but to be human.

Carl G. Jung, *Man and His Symbols*

It is in the whole process of meeting and solving problems that life has meaning. Problems are the cutting edge that distinguishes between success and failure. Problems call forth our courage and our wisdom; indeed, they create our courage and our wisdom. It is only because of problems that we grow mentally and spiritually. It is through the pain of confronting and resolving problems that we learn.

M. Scott Peck, *The Road Less Traveled*

Contents

List of Illustrations	ix
Acknowledgments	xii
Introduction	xiv

CHAPTER 1 History and Formulation ... 1
Brief History ... 1
Transition to Kentucky and Development of the American
 Art Therapy Association ... 5

CHAPTER 2 Media Dimension Variables ... 8

CHAPTER 3 Theoretical Structure ... 13
Basic Foundations of the Expressive Therapies Continuum (ETC) ... 13
Entrainment, Resonance, and Isomorphism ... 16
Processing and Evaluating Response to Media Properties ... 17
Actions and Metaphors ... 18
Boundaries and Cognition ... 19
Symbolic Representation and Interpretation ... 20
Integration of Concepts ... 20

CHAPTER 4 Kinesthetic-/Sensory-Focused Initiatives ... 23
Introduction to the Clinical Practice Guide ... 23
Initiative One—Scribble Chase Mural ... 24
Initiative Two—Expressions in Movement and Sound ... 29
Initiative Three—Media Properties and Range of Materials ... 34
Initiative Four—Visual Breathing ... 38

CHAPTER 5 Perceptual-/Affective-Focused Initiatives ... 45
Initiative Five—Expressive Drawings: Mind States—Mood States ... 46
Initiative Six—Dyadic Nonverbal Communication ... 53
Initiative Seven—How I See Myself/How Others See Me ... 57
Initiative Eight—Haptic/Visual Self Symbol ... 60
Initiative Nine—Changing Points of View 1 ... 65
Initiative Ten—Images of Pain and Healing ... 71
Initiative Eleven—Mandala, the Great Round ... 76

CHAPTER 6 Cognitive-/Symbolic-Focused Initiatives	88
Initiative Twelve—The Word	89
Initiative Thirteen—Changing Points of View 2	92
Introduction to Guided Imagery	95
Initiative Fourteen—Guided Imagery—The Source	97
Initiative Fifteen—Guided Imagery—The Dwelling	101
Initiative Sixteen—Guided Imagery—The Cave	106
Initiative Seventeen—Environmental Awareness	111
Initiative Eighteen—Box Self (Inner/Outer Self)	115
Initiative Nineteen—Body Tracing	118
Initiative Twenty—Lifeline	121
Initiative Twenty-One—12 Archetypes and My Roles in Life	126
My Roles in Life	128
Initiative Twenty-Two—Persona Masks—Anima and Animus: the Shadow Self	130
Initiative Twenty-Three—Battle Drawing	134
Initiative Twenty-Four—Powerful and Powerless Collage	137
Initiative Twenty-Five—Rhyne's Problem-Solving Collage	141
Initiative Twenty-Six—Family-of-Origin Sculpture	145
Initiative Twenty-Seven—Survival on an Island	148
Initiative Twenty-Eight—The Bridge (Bridge the Opposites)	154
CHAPTER 7 Creativity and Its Role	159
Data Management, Brain Flow, and Resolution	160
Resonance and Resolution	164
Education and Creativity	165
Art and Creativity	167
Conclusion	175
Appendix 1: Additional References	177
Appendix 2: Resources	179
Index	180

Illustrations

Color Figures

4.3 Visual Breathing
4.4 Visual Breathing
4.5 Visual Breathing
4.6 Visual Breathing
5.1 Expressive Drawings: Mind States—Mood States (Mad)
5.2 Expressive Drawings: Mind States—Mood States (Sad)
5.3 Expressive Drawings: Mind States—Mood States (Glad)
5.4 Expressive Drawings: Mind States—Mood States (Scared)
5.7 How I See Myself
5.8 How Others See Me
5.12 Changing Points of View 1 (Painting 1)
5.13 Changing Points of View 1 (Close-up)
5.14 Changing Points of View 1 (Painting 2)
5.15 Changing Points of View 1 (Painting 3)
5.16 Images of Pain and Healing (Image of Pain)
5.17 Images of Pain and Healing (Image of Healing)
5.18 Images of Pain and Healing (Image of Healing Integrating with Pain)
5.19 Mandala, the Great Round
5.20 Mandala, the Great Round
5.21 Mandala, the Great Round
5.22 Mandala, the Great Round
5.23 Mandala, the Great Round
5.24 Mandala, the Great Round
5.25 Mandala, the Great Round
5.26 Mandala, the Great Round
6.2 Changing Points of View 2 (Painting 1)
6.3 Changing Points of View 2 (Enlarge a Section)
6.4 Changing Points of View 2 (Painting 3)
6.5 Guided Imagery—The Source
6.6 Guided Imagery—The Source
6.10 Guided Imagery—The Cave
6.11 Guided Imagery—The Cave
6.12 Guided Imagery—The Cave
6.13 Environmental Awareness

6.15 Box Self (Inner/Outer Self)
6.20 Persona Masks
6.21 Persona Masks
6.22 Battle Drawing
6.23 Powerful and Powerless Collage (Powerful)
6.24 Powerful and Powerless Collage (Powerless)
6.25 Rhyne's Problem-Solving Collage
6.26 Family Sculpture
6.29 The Bridge (Bridge the Opposites)
6.30 The Bridge (Bridge the Opposites)

Figures

4.1	Scribble Chase Mural	26
4.2	Expressions in Movement and Sound	31
4.3	Visual Breathing	39
4.4	Visual Breathing	40
4.5	Visual Breathing	41
4.6	Visual Breathing	42
4.7	Visual Breathing	42
5.1	Expressive Drawings: Mind States—Mood States (Mad)	49
5.2	Expressive Drawings: Mind States—Mood States (Sad)	49
5.3	Expressive Drawings: Mind States—Mood States (Glad)	50
5.4	Expressive Drawings: Mind States—Mood States (Scared)	50
5.5	Dyadic Nonverbal Communication	54
5.6	Dyadic Nonverbal Communication	55
5.7	How I See Myself	58
5.8	How Others See Me	58
5.9	Haptic-Visual Self Symbol	61
5.10	Haptic-Visual Self Symbol	61
5.11	Haptic-Visual Self Symbol	63
5.12	Changing Points of View 1 (Painting 1)	66
5.13	Changing Points of View 1 (Close-up)	66
5.14	Changing Points of View 1 (Painting 2)	67
5.15	Changing Points of View 1 (Painting 3)	67
5.16	Images of Pain and Healing (Image of Pain)	72
5.17	Images of Pain and Healing (Image of Healing)	73
5.18	Images of Pain and Healing (Image of Healing Integrating with Pain)	74
5.19	Mandala, the Great Round	77
5.20	Mandala, the Great Round	79
5.21	Mandala, the Great Round	83
5.22	Mandala, the Great Round	83

5.23	Mandala, the Great Round	84
5.24	Mandala, the Great Round	84
5.25	Mandala, the Great Round	85
5.26	Mandala, the Great Round	85
6.1	The Word	90
6.2	Changing Points of View 2 (Painting 1)	93
6.3	Changing Points of View 2 (Enlarge a Section)	93
6.4	Changing Points of View 2 (Painting 3)	94
6.5	Guided Imagery—The Source	99
6.6	Guided Imagery—The Source	99
6.7	Guided Imagery—Dwelling	103
6.8	Guided Imagery—Dwelling	103
6.9	Guided Imagery—Dwelling	104
6.10	Guided Imagery—The Cave	107
6.11	Guided Imagery—The Cave	108
6.12	Guided Imagery—The Cave	108
6.13	Environmental Awareness	112
6.14	Box Self (Inner/Outer Self)	116
6.15	Box Self (Inner/Outer Self)	116
6.16	Body Tracing	119
6.17	Lifeline	122
6.18	Lifeline	123
6.19	My Roles in Life and the 12 Archetypes	129
6.20	Persona Masks	131
6.21	Persona Masks	131
6.22	Battle Drawing	135
6.23	Powerful and Powerless Collage (Powerful)	138
6.24	Powerful and Powerless Collage (Powerless)	138
6.25	Rhyne's Problem-Solving Collage	142
6.26	Family Sculpture	146
6.27	Survival on an Island	150
6.28	Survival on an Island	151
6.29	The Bridge (Bridge the Opposites)	155
6.30	The Bridge (Bridge the Opposites)	156

Tables

3.1	Relationship of ETC to Graphic and Play Development	20
3.2	Media Dimension Variables	21

Box

4.1	Rating Scale for MDV Lab	36

Acknowledgments

As one of the pioneers and a founding member of the American Art Therapy Association, I dedicate this book to the unfailing energy that developed our profession. Not only to those "pioneers" and "early settlers" but also to the current generation, and generations to come, of scientist-artists who understand the integration of the two.

I also thank my coauthor, who has worked tirelessly on this project while rearing teenagers and a younger child, serving as chair of an expanding university department, and being a great partner to my son.

As I look back on my life, I realize I lived in a wonderful era and atmosphere in which creativity and innovation flourished. I am blessed with an incredible family, and I love my life. This journey has been fun!

Sandra (Kagin) Graves-Alcorn

The last words are the most difficult and the most important:

Thank you, Sandra, for inviting me into this endeavor with you. I am flattered and honored to be sharing this book and this experience with you. You have been such a significant figure in my life. Your love of this profession is energizing, your knowledge is vast, and your joy is contagious!

Second, I must thank my students who teach me as I teach them and who have so graciously shared their art and their experiences with us for this text. Without them, it would not be possible. You are all wonderful!

Thank you to Clare and Jenny for the hours of editing, assisting, and support during this endeavor. I am proud to call you colleagues and blessed to call you friends.

Thank you to my parents, who have always loved and supported me and prepared me for this accomplishment.

Finally, I want to thank my family for their support and grace. They have tolerated long hours away, leftovers for dinner AGAIN! and my exhaustion. To Ethan, Maren, and Abby—you are my sunshine and my heart, and I love you so much! You are the best kids in the world! To Stephen, my loving husband, best friend, and number-one fan—your belief in me and support of my work astound me. I love you, and I am so blessed to have you in my life. And last but most importantly, I am who I am, because I have been saved by Jesus, and I am eternally grateful!

Christa Kagin

Introduction

This book introduces the practitioner and/or student to the Expressive Therapies Continuum and explains the Media Dimension Variables (ETC-MDV). It is a thorough discussion of the history, framework, and application of the ETC-MDV. It includes the original initiatives used at its inception and newer initiatives that have been repeatedly used in therapeutic practice. Detailed directives, materials used, and therapeutic goals are presented. The authors also provide therapeutic transitions, adaptations, and creativity activation for each initiative. These initiatives make for a user-friendly, hands-on manual for a variety of practitioners in mental health as well as a great text for teaching students of art therapy. The material in this manual is presented for successful application by readers in all fields.

CHAPTER 1

History and Formulation

Sandra (Kagin) Graves-Alcorn

In the year 1964, I began a sojourn that was to last the rest of my life and, with the writing of this book, hopefully beyond. I am also delighted that a second generation of Kagin art therapists has joined me in this endeavor. Christa Pickens was a graduate student of mine at the University of Louisville, where she met my son Stephen Kagin. She is now my daughter-in-law! I am proud that she also took the academic route and is associate professor and chair of the Art Department at Benedictine College in Atchison, Kansas. Christa and Stephen also gave me three wonderful grandchildren!

Brief History

We believe history is very important to critical thinking and creativity. It is essential to know what went before and what kind of thinking went into change.

This history is from my own experience as I remember it.

In 1964, while at the University of Tulsa completing my B.A. in Fine Arts, I was fortunate to be in a child psychology class taught by Dr. Robert Parrish. Early in the semester, Dr. Parrish mentioned the term "art therapy" and said there was an art therapist at the Children's Memorial Center. I was so excited, as I had been wondering if art could be used in psychology and healing. After class, I told the professor that I wanted to study art therapy, and he set up an independent apprenticeship with Margaret Howard at the Children's Memorial Center.

Marge was a feisty, enthusiastic, and funny woman in her 60s. She had been sent to New York to take classes in art therapy with Margaret Naumburg, the acknowledged American pioneer of our profession. In New York, she had met Elinor Ulman, Elsie Mueller, and Irene Jakab, all of whom later played a huge role in my professional life.

Marge worked at an in-patient hospital for children and adolescents who were diagnosed as severely emotionally disturbed or schizophrenic. Those were the days long before the American Psychiatric Association's *Diagnostic and Statistical Manual of Mental Disorders*. The youth were in long-term care that was psychodynamic in orientation. This was where I completed my apprenticeship with Marge and where I would begin the real first steps of my journey. I shall always be grateful to this lovely lady, who shared her information with me and led me to ask questions and develop my own answers, as well as reference many others in leading the trek across the professional and academic plains of art therapy.

Marge began by reading her notes from Naumburg's class then allowed me to observe her working with a patient. She had a large art room, fully stocked with materials, and she saw both individuals and groups. After about a week, I was introduced to my first patient. The girl was just a bit younger than I and taught me a great lesson in manipulation and transference/countertransference. She was doing a painting when she informed me that she was running away and wanted me to promise not to tell. I could not have been more green and naïve! Fortunately, I disclosed this bit of information with Marge, who laughed and told me I had been "had"!

One of my favorite stories about Marge was that during World War II, she had earned a living painting nudes on cigarettes. I realized this was one creative woman who was way ahead of her time! Years later, as I reflect on that experience, I realize that the creativity of the therapist is so essential that it cannot be separated from the clinician; rather, it is part of the art therapist's success.

At the end of the year, I graduated and set out to establish myself as an art therapist. In 1965, I was hired by the Hissom Memorial Center in Sand Springs, Oklahoma, as a social worker in the department of psychology, as there was no classification for an art therapist. I also started my master's degree in special education and child psychology.

Hissom was a state facility for what was then called the mentally retarded, although many of the residents would have been diagnosed differently today. The "children" (some were adults, but we called them all children back then) were divided by IQ and level of adaptive functioning and lived in cottages together. There was also a large infirmary that housed individuals with severe hydrocephalus, phenylketonuria (PKU), brain damage, and other debilitating injuries and illnesses. At that time, they were called the "profoundly retarded." This unit was very difficult for me to even walk into, and there was no art therapy in there. (It would be several years before the sensory operant stimulation [SOS] movement would arrive here and in other similar units.)

Children were brought to me in a room in the psychology department. They were called "the worst of the worst," and I shall never forget them. My first published article was about a 9-year-old named Becky and entitled "Art Therapy with Atypical Retarded Children." I presented this research at the founding meeting of the American Society of Psychopathology of Expression in Washington, DC. It was there that I met Irene Jakab and Elinor Ulman. Irene became a personal friend and mentor.

Elinor Ulman studied with Margaret Naumburg at New York University and became an artist-therapist at a hospital in Washington, DC. She was the first publisher and editor of *Bulletin of Art in Psychotherapy, Education and Rehabilitation*. Her "art as therapy" approach emphasized the intrinsic therapeutic potential in the art-making process and the central role the defense mechanism of sublimation plays in this experience. Ulman's most outstanding contributions to the field have been as an editor and writer. She was also on the ad hoc committee that wrote the bylaws to develop the American Art Therapy Association. She founded *Bulletin of Art Therapy* in 1961 (*American Journal of Art Therapy* after 1970) when no other publication of its kind existed. Elinor was a woman way ahead of her time. In her youth, she interned with Frank Lloyd Wright. She fought hard to get this position then was relegated to the kitchen! In 1983, she nominated me as president of the American Art Therapy Association, telling me, "I believe you have the seasoned intelligence to do the job." My last memory of Elinor was lovely. She and I, along with Robin Goodman (also a past president), had visited Elinor at her home in Vermont. It was just a few years prior to her death in 1991 and we were literally sitting on the dock of her "golden pond," laughing with the sun on our backs.

These two powerful, pioneering women became not only my mentors but also my role models, and I remain grateful to this day for their encouragement.

The founding meeting of the American Society of Psychopathology of Expression in 1965 in Washington, DC, brought together some of the best-known psychiatrists and psychologists of the day. This organization preceded the American Art Therapy Association and was a stellar gathering of scholars and practitioners. It was held at the National Gallery of Art and hosted by Dr. Raymond Stites, noted author and expert on the sublimations of Leonardo da Vinci. I was to present my first professional paper at the American Association of the Psychopathology of Expression . . . and I was terrified! My presentation was terrible, but I was forgiven for my youth. Although I had written the thing out, I tried to talk extemporaneously. I will never forget Elinor Ulman coming up to me and saying, "No matter what you said I see tremendous potential in you!" (This paper was published in *Psychiatry and Art*, 1968 and entitled "Psychiatric Art Therapy with Atypical Retarded Children.")

Having been taught the principles of psychodynamically oriented art therapy, which relies on the projection of unconscious material to gain insight, I quickly became lost in treating these children at Hissom, as insight was not a realistic goal due to their level of cognitive functioning. I began studying cognitive and developmental psychology and learned which art materials were appropriate for treatment of this population and which were not.

In 1967, I obtained the position of director of art and occupational therapy at Parsons State Hospital in Parsons, Kansas. This research facility was well-funded with grants studying adaptive behavior of the mentally retarded. I met and worked with Dr. Henry Leland. In fact, Henry introduced me to my first husband.

It began to occur to me that the appropriate "therapy" to use with the "mentally retarded" (and so too with any population) was directly related to the media, the project, and the structure of the sessions. Most sessions were done in large groups, covering all ranges of what was then called mental retardation from severe to borderline.

I had an incredible staff and budget. The team had our own building, with large studio space as well as private therapy rooms. My budget for just art supplies was more than $5,000! It is hard to imagine what this translates to in today's market.

My colleagues were artists and very creative. We studied what seemed to "work" with the various groups and individuals. I was also completing my master's degree at that time, so I applied what I had developed programmatically into fairly sophisticated variable definitions and statistics. The concept of Media Dimension Variables (MDV) was born.

Transition to Kentucky and Development of the American Art Therapy Association

Through my friend Bob Ault (later to be original president-elect of the American Art Therapy Association [AATA] and then president), I sought a contact in Kentucky, because at this time I was married, and my husband wanted to attend law school near his family, and this required a move. He told me that a Dr. Roger White had started an art therapy master's degree at the University of Louisville. I did contact Dr. White, who told me that the program was defunct but still on the books and asked if I would like to start one (very different world in hiring back then)!

Simultaneously, several people had formed an ad hoc committee to develop a professional organization, and serendipity took over, as that founding meeting was scheduled at the University of Louisville in June of 1969, the same day I was interviewed to become a faculty member. The ad hoc committee consisted of Myra Levick, Bob Ault, Elinor Ulman, Don Jones, and Felice Cohen.

I have absolutely wonderful memories of these people, and if the purpose of this book were to delve deeply into the history of the American Art Therapy Association, founded that hot June day of 1969, it would be a volume of material. I will mention, however, that on that day, we passed and adopted the bylaws of the American Art Therapy Association. Myra Levick (Hahnemann College) was elected president and Bob Ault president-elect (Menninger Foundation). Don Jones (Harding Hospital) was secretary and Marge Howard (Children's Medical Center) was treasurer. I was elected chair of education (highly qualified, since an hour earlier I had just been hired by the University of Louisville!), Ben Ploger (Louisiana) was standards chair, Elsie Mueller (Kansas) was parliamentarian, and Helen Landgarten (California) was public relations chair. All these individuals contributed greatly to the field of art therapy and are considered the professional pioneers and should be familiar to anyone who has studied in this field. At the date of this writing, only two of us are still alive, me and Myra Levick, the last of the original pioneers. That was also the day I discovered I was pregnant with my first child, who 28 years later met and married my coauthor!

Through the years, the concepts of Media Dimension Variables were further studied and refined. I joined the faculty of the University of Louisville in 1969 to revamp and resurrect a master's degree in art therapy, which had begun in 1956, graduated two students, then lay dormant since 1957. I was able to develop a course of study that included my theoretical background and experiences and promoted the efficacy of both art as therapy and art psychotherapy. In fact, I saw this well-worn argument by other professionals as a continuum of interventions, allowing flexibility and including a wide range of populations who could benefit from art therapists' services.

One of my hopes for this book is the realization that together as expressive arts therapists, we are stronger and have more influence to make a difference in health care.

In the early 1970s, I founded the Institute of Expressive Therapies with the intent to include music, dance, drama, and poetry in the curriculum of the master's degree in expressive therapies. This was the beginning of art therapists observing the commonalities rather than the differences among the disciplines. It has long been my contention that the creative arts therapies together have a professional foundation that differentiates us from all other mental health professionals. The Expressive Therapies Summit, held each November in New York City, was founded by Barry Cohen during his role as executive director of Expressive Media, Inc. (Judy Rubin and Ellie Irwin formed this organization in the mid-1980s, and I was asked to join the executive board in 2011.) The success of this endeavor and its cutting-edge mission of integration of the healing arts may be what ultimately defines and saves our profession. At the writing of this book, there are few stand-alone masters' programs in art therapy. Most have been subsumed into counseling curricula.

When my colleague Vija Lusebrink joined the faculty, we researched the interrelationship among the various expressive therapies, later to culminate in our published article "The Expressive Therapies Continuum" in 1978. We found a commonality first in developmental theory. The well-known work of Viktor Lowenfeld (1957) in the field of art education had been one of the foundations of MDV. Since the field of art therapy was fixing "deviating" behaviors, then what was the expected "normal" or expected and acceptable behavior in the arts arena? To recognize deviations, one must know the developmental norms. Although other researchers wrote about the development of children's graphic expression, I was especially taken with Lowenfeld, as he fit with my other favorite developmentalist, Jean Piaget. When the stages were placed side by side, they beautifully explained each other.

References

Graves, S. (1968). Psychiatric art therapy with atypical retarded children. In Jakab, I. (Ed.), *Psychiatry and Art: Proceedings of the IVth International Colloquium of Psychopathology of Expression*, pp. 68–74. Basel, NY: Karger Press.

Lowenfeld, V. (1957). *Creative and Mental Growth* (3rd ed.). New York, NY: MacMillan.

CHAPTER 2

Media Dimension Variables

Sandra Graves-Alcorn

The concept of exploring variables in use of media was the subject of my master's thesis. The following has been quoted in numerous articles, the latest being my chapter in the book *Expressive Arts and Play Therapy with Children and Adolescents* (Green and Drews, 2014).

Exploitation of media dimension variables, those qualities or properties inherent in a given medium and process which may be utilized in a therapeutic or educational situation to evaluate and/or elicit a desired response from an individual.

(Kagin, 1969)

The premises upon which the concept of media dimension variables (MDV) was developed are:

1. The reinforcement value of making "art" can be a therapeutic process;
2. All individuals can be creative to some degree;
3. Dimensions of art media are discernible and can be classified; and
4. Media dimensions can be therapeutically applied.

(Kagin, 1969)

The numerous definitions of creativity back then were focused on behavior change and later on information system retrieval to develop unique thoughts. In the early years of its professional development, art therapy focused on the projections of unconscious material, directed toward the goal of insight into inner conflicts. Little attention was given to the media by which these projections were promoted. I therefore began looking at specific properties of art media and attempted to hypothesize general emotional or other behavioral responses.

The physical properties of media such as fluidity, malleability, indestructibility, expansiveness, unpredictability, adaptability, and other factors that will be better defined later were explored. Three generalized variables were delineated: **structure**, **task complexity**, and **media properties**. The following is taken directly from my thesis to explain these variables as understood in 1969:

I. Structure
   A. Task directions—range from prescribing precise use of materials toward a preconceived product end to very limited explanation of purpose (example; difference between an origami project and handing the individual paint and brush for a "free-expressive" (doing anything you wish with this) task.
   B. Material manipulation—structure can be inextricably related to qualities and/or quantities of materials or entirely apart from the media properties.
   C. Environmental or behavior boundaries—expectations within the building and therapeutic situation are upheld by some method of control and/or conditioning. It is believed that, although art can be an intrinsic motivator and reward or a means of aiding alleviation of emotional distress, there are many times when behavior which prohibits use of intrinsic resources must be controlled extrinsically. The hyperactive, highly agitated, distractible, emotionally volatile individual cannot receive much benefit from an activity to which he is not attending or in which he is not participating. Operant procedures have been utilized with several patients in individual therapy to help them contain such behaviors.

II. Complexity
   The difficulty of a given task in terms of the number of operations necessary for execution and completion and the dexterity required to carry through with the operations are assessed in terms of the cognitive development and capabilities of the individual. Repetition of an operation (such as pounding 20 nails instead of one) was not considered to be a factor in complexity.

III. Physical Properties
Materials are soft or hard, fluid or solidified, smooth or rough in texture, large or small, etc. Obviously, these properties are not dichotomized, but range in **a continuum**.

(Kagin, 1969)

Combinations of complexity, structure, and media properties elicited six potential classifications of art projects: high and low complexity, structured and unstructured, fluid media and resistive media. Each project was thus designated as **HC** (high complexity, which randomly assigned three steps and more for definition) and **LC** (low complexity which entailed fewer than three steps for completion of the project), **U** (unstructured, meaning nondirected) and **S** (structured, meaning having specific directions), and **F** (fluid media) to **R** (resistive media).

Media whose properties were soft, aqueous, malleable, and easy to manipulate, such as finger paint, soft clay, or polymer acrylics, were in the fluid range. Resistive materials were defined as hard, brittle, slightly pliable to nonmalleable, and difficult to manipulate, such as hard or highly grogged clay, metal, wood, poster boards, heavier papers, or pencils (Green and Drews, 2014). After observing working with many clients over the years and ascertaining what appeared to be successful for them, I chose three or more sequential steps to be considered high complexity, and I ascribed low complexity when only one or two steps were required.

The directions given for the task were divided into structured and unstructured projects. The unstructured projects had goals for completion that were left up to the individual, and the instructions were simple, as in: "Paint anything you wish" or "Put the metal on the board in any design you like." The structured task was very specific on how to use the materials and what the end result should be, such as "use these pictures to make a collage that represents your family" or "draw a house." I applied these principles to the population at the Parsons State Hospital in Parsons, Kansas. I divided our programs into several segments in order to serve as much of the population as possible. The lower-functioning residents were in the art behavior reinforcement group. They were given a sorting task, which was timed, each day. If they beat the time from the previous day, they were rewarded with an art experience. These experiences were very simple and assisted by the staff. Experiences such as finger paint printing, polymer tissue collages, found-object stamp art, splatter paint, and straw blowing were used. The residents were delighted with the activity and the results. We always framed or matted all or part of the group work and put it on the walls or easels until the next week's sessions.

The second grouping of residents (developmental art group) relied on levels of graphic development at either the preschematic or schematic levels (Lowenfeld, 1957). Members of this group were given a variety of activities that reinforced development of patterns, problem solving, or expression of emotion. Most of these residents functioned at the moderate to mild level of retardation and adaptive behavior (American Association of the Mentally Deficient terminology in 1965).

A third group (the "psychiatric" group) were residents with serious acting-out problems, and they were typically seen individually in a separate therapy room. I planned interventions for each based on the assessment and the treatment plan developed by the treatment team, which consisted of psychologists, psychiatrists, social workers, the cottage life coordinator, a music therapist, and me.

The fourth group was entitled "Socialization and Self-Image" and consisted of the higher-functioning residents. Group work on body image and presentation of self in public were the rationale for these residents. The goal at that time was for the resident to be "invisible" in the mainstream. Matching colors and fabrics for clothing and communicating with each other in nonverbal dyads they drew and then discussed their drawings. It introduced them to some art history and famous paintings which helped residents relate to each other on a personal level.

These programs were enormously successful, and just before I left Parsons State Hospital, I developed an art show that was placed in a local bank, exhibiting the residents' work, and hosted an opening to which people from the community were invited. It was called "A Special Child's View" and was very well received.

Today, these media dimension variables have been expanded in scope, as they were integrated into the expressive therapies continuum. Our understanding of creativity, mindfulness, and brain function, all of which will be discussed later, has given more and more validity to the original ideas and hypotheses. Now we have a richness of data from which the initiatives in this book have been developed and utilized. Years of clinical experience also lend efficacy to my original youthful enthusiasm, and I am grateful that both MDV and ETC have stood the test of time.

References

Green, E., and Drews, A. (Eds.) (2014). *Integrating Expressive Arts and Play Therapy with Children and Adolescents*. Hoboken, NJ: Wiley.

Kagin, S. (1969). *The Influence of Structure in Painting on Verbal and Graphic Self-Expression of Retarded Youth*. Unpublished Master's Thesis, University of Tulsa.

Lowenfeld, V. (1957). *Creative and Mental Growth* (3rd ed.). New York, NY: MacMillan.

CHAPTER 3

Theoretical Structure

Basic Foundations of the Expressive Therapies Continuum (ETC)

Practical application of the Expressive Therapies Continuum depends on the understanding of the definitions used, a working knowledge of historical concepts related to the development of creative capacities, and sound psychological understanding. We begin this chapter, then, with definitions and theory related to the ETC and its developmental structure. The definitions of the variables in the continuum are as follows, derived from the *Merriam-Webster Dictionary of the English Language* (2015):

- Kinesthetic: "relating to the use of sense organs in your muscles and other body parts to feel the position and movements of your body."
- Sensory: "relating to sensation, to the perception of a stimulus, to the voyage made by incoming nerve impulses from the sense organs to the nerve centers or to the senses themselves."
- Perceptual: "relating to, or involving perception (the ability to see, hear, or become aware of something through the senses) especially in relation to immediate sensory experience."
- Affective: "relating to, arising from, or influencing feelings or emotions: emotional, cognitive and affective symptoms."
- Cognitive: "relating to, or involving conscious mental activities (such as thinking, understanding, learning, and remembering)."
- Symbolic: "expressing or representing an idea or quality without using words; relating to or being used as a symbol; using symbols."

A seventh term, "creativity," originally included as one of the ETC levels, will be discussed in its own chapter.

Our work on the ETC makes use of developmental theories of Jean Piaget and Victor Lowenfeld, who were strong influences in the development of our strategies and initiatives. The development of *schemata* in particular was of common importance to both Piaget and Lowenfeld as a pattern of thinking that built upon itself and manifested in drawing behaviors, play behaviors, and the development of symbolic language.

Piaget's developmental sequences (sensorimotor play, preoperational play, and concrete operational and formal operational thinking) provide a helpful framework for describing and selecting various arts and experiences: properties of the media, structure (control), and complexity (cognitive understanding) of the task (initiative).

Sensorimotor play, in which the infant and toddler acquire knowledge through movement and practice play, translates here into the **Kinesthetic/Sensory** level of the continuum. Practice play begins at birth, as babies repeat motions over and over until the action is assimilated and accommodated and a lifelong striving toward homeostasis is set in motion. Sometimes, for whatever reason, we get stuck in a kinesthetic pattern and perseveration takes place. In adults, these patterns can take the form of rituals, habits, manners of speech, and even lifestyles. Often in therapy we need to return to a kinesthetic sensorimotor state to break the patterns and create a new form of adaptation. In current literature, this ability is often referred to as **resiliency**.

The **Perceptual/Affective level** begins as motion becomes form and as touch or other sensory experiences affect feelings. These feelings may be reptilian brain functions (such as the sensation of being startled) and are not yet part of operational thought, but they do begin to activate the connecting limbic function with which they are associated. Emotions have a survival function. They can release adrenaline to create **anger**, which enables us to make change in the immediate present. **Sadness** slows down the body and mind to prepare us to process loss. **Fear** alerts us to danger, and **happiness** or joy balances all the other experiences and gives us motivation for growth and resilience. As these physical manifestations begin to develop further into signs, symbols, and other facets of language (operational thinking), a meaning becomes attached to the action that created the form, and the **Cognitive/Symbolic level** is attained.

The stages of Graphic Development that were developed by Viktor Lowenfeld may be aligned with Piaget's development of a schemata, or a pattern of thinking upon which we all build throughout a lifetime. Lowenfeld also described "schema" as a visual pattern of rules resulting from early scribble behavior to making concentric movements to attaining control enough to create form and name it (Lowenfeld and Brittain, 1970, 1987).

The first stage, the action of various types of scribbles (entitled the Scribble Stage), is a form of practice play that evolves from strokes to concentric loops and then into closed form. This stage can begin at around 12 to 18 months, and the movements are random in nature. Scribbling is a sensorimotor activity that defines figure and ground on the paper (or whatever the child chooses as recipient of the action). In this stage, the motion is more important than the mark. As will be identified and applied in the initiatives later in this book, the use of scribbling assists in the regression process, first as tapping or marking the field and then, when longitudinal scribbling begins around age 2, as focusing on experimenting with linear and circular motion. When these motions are mastered, around age 3, the form is purposely constructed and often named. Here we see the beginning of symbolic play and preschematic form, and the encephalopod (body/head configuration) is born. This occurs at approximately ages 3 to 4, and the ability to draw a human figure begins (Kagin, 1978).

In the preschematic stage (around ages 4 to 6), much practice and change take place. A child's forms do not yet have a set pattern and may represent several things to him or her. The forms are usually randomly placed on the page. When a schema develops (about age 6 or 7), the child has established a definite pattern or set of rules for drawing objects or people. As operational thinking develops, so do the drawings. A tree or house or person is drawn in the same general style until the child has an experience significant enough to trigger a deviation from the schema. This is also the time period when symbolic play becomes both liquidating and/or compensating a significant event. In liquidating play, the child may destroy a love object (something symbolic of the loss), reenacting a death or major loss. At the same time, the child may use compensatory play, resurrecting the loss or reuniting the family or giving love where abuse actually occurred (Piaget, 1962).

The drawings of children in the preschematic and schematic ranges of development are so powerful and full of information that they are often used in the courts by an expert witness art therapist in abuse, trauma, or custody cases. Although not within the scope and purpose of this book, it is vital for any caregivers to be aware of the expected drawing behaviors of young children—as these may be the first indicators of a problem—and then take any concerns to a professional.

The Realistic Stage begins when children attempt to draw what they see rather than the concept of what they perceive. Realism arises around the age of nine and corresponds to the development of operational thinking, when logic may be used and children begin to understand their thinking is unique to them.

Naturalism is the next stage, which yields an exploration of abstract ideas and represents not only the object or scene but the emotional valence attached to the environment.

Entrainment, Resonance, and Isomorphism

How do media enhance or inhibit this development? It is by processes of **entrainment**, **resonance**, and **isomorphism** that the media affect the motion and the amount of physical, mental or emotional energy needed to elicit kinesthetic, emotional, and intellectual resources. In a review of the psychological effects of brainwave entrainment (BWE), Huang and Charyton (2008) describe it as the use of rhythmic stimuli with the intention of producing a frequency-following response (resonance) of brainwaves to match the frequency of the stimuli (p. 38). Resonance thus is found at the perceptual level, even though its beginnings may be sensorimotor. The stimuli, here speaking about the properties of the arts media, must command a focusing to adjust the brainwaves to a level of resonance. If an individual finds pleasure (positive reinforcement value) in the use of a medium, then motivation to continue is present, allowing the media stimuli to connect with brain frequencies (alpha) associated with light sleep, creativity and insight. Beta frequencies, which are associated with thinking and focusing, may also be reached as the resonance deepens into an isomorphic state. It is also important to note the sensitivity to resonance produced by media properties and perceptual activity. A high beta response is associated with intensity or anxiety and can be brought about by using media with a very negative reinforcement value or by using the media in a manner contraindicated by its liquid- or solid-state properties.

The expressive arts therapists, therefore, need to be keenly aware of the interaction between the material and the person. When structure and complexity are added to this matrix, we observe a shift in cognitive functioning that includes verbal skills, nonverbal skills, memory, attention, and general intelligence. Although Huang reviewed data related primarily to auditory and visual light stimuli, we have extrapolated to include more media variants. The work of David Siegel further explains these mental processes as interrelated aspects of the energy and information flow. He describes mental processes (moods to thoughts) as parts of a spectrum of a state of mind in any given moment. Siegel (2012) studies mental life, which includes an intentional focus of attention, the directing of energy, and information flow, which shapes neural firing in the brain as much as neural firing shapes attention! Through the use of the ETC and its MDV, we can elicit, expose, and direct a focus of attention and redirect the flow of energy and information. We contend that this leads to a neuroplasticity that fosters resilience in life.

In more simple terms, think now of other arts and play forms—such as movement and dance, sound and music, sand play, "pretend" play, or drama. These forms follow the same development on the continuum. If isomorphism takes place and the individual becomes attuned to the media, with a clear understanding of the structure (direction), then some emotional response should be elicited. We can then help the student or client compartmentalize the emotions and deal with each separately rather than be overwhelmed by experiencing all at once.

Processing and Evaluating Response to Media Properties

The assessment component of a project or experience is very valuable. Practitioners will want to ask several questions of the student or client. Do the materials resonate with the person? If not, explore why. There are several possibilities why resonance did not occur. For example, the materials may not have been of sufficient quality to enable a full experience of the activity. Poor-quality materials can be very frustrating. If you have ever tried to finger paint on drawing paper without water, then you understand why you do not want to try that again. Runny paints on paper set on an easel can be upsetting. Modeling clay often does not substitute for the real thing. Test materials before you buy or use them, or you will feel like a surgeon stitching a wound with rope and resonance will not occur. If you have quality materials, however, it is a study in temperament whether the person discovers resonance or resistance. Certain sensory experiences can set a person "on edge" and have an aversive reaction. This happens frequently with different types of clay, for example. The action upon the materials may also tap into deep unconscious experiences that were unpleasant. Previous experience with the materials also comes into play here.

Actions and Metaphors

Materials create action and reaction and enhance awareness of body, mind, and spirit. Materials can be experienced metaphorically and describe how we feel—smooth, sticky, rough, sharp, slippery, and so forth. They create a positive or negative sensation and have a reinforcement value for each individual from none to high arousal.

Fluid materials generally elicit a "loose," flowing response that is usually pleasant. Pleasurable experiences motivate the individual to continue their use and are defined as having a high or good reinforcement value. Watercolor markers, prevalent in therapy and classes, have a built in "mediator" in that although the color is fluid, the container can be controlled. Finger paints, however, are literally "hands on" and tend to elicit a "messy" look, which can be unpleasant for some people and therefore of low reinforcement value.

Therapists/practitioners should help the individual to resonate with the flow rather than the look of the materials first. Ask for a description of the experience, such as "smearing" or "smoothing." Explain that the words used to describe the experience may be metaphors for their own emotional or cognitive life. The terms the individual uses to describe the experience may lead to recall of past events, which will assist in gaining insight. What does the term "smearing" evoke? What does the term "smoothing" evoke? Ask the person to use as many words as possible to describe the experience. These metaphors may be explored immediately or in later work. Talking about the medium as a component of the self may be introduced here, allowing the student or client to be aware of his or her uniqueness and the "aliveness" of the art experience rather than trying to make something "pretty." This kind of discussion also helps with the "I can't draw a straight line" phrase with which we are all familiar! Get judgment and the cognitive out of the head straight on.

When she introduced Gestalt art therapy in 1974, Janie Rhyne approached what she called the "process as the self" (Rhyne, 1974) and asked her clients to give the experience (drawing, painting, clay) a voice, preceding a description of materials, line, form, color, space with "I am." This kind of exercise reinforces the resonance with the materials and can have quite startling results.

Boundaries and Cognition

Boundaries define a space, set limits, and create the ability to function. We all need boundaries to maintain a social stance and personal safety. Behavior that is appropriate usually adheres to a standard of the boundary, while behaviors that are inappropriate can go "astray," create havoc, and lack direction. Our media may be defined as *quantity* determined or *boundary* determined (Kagin and Lusebrink, 1978). A piece of wood is boundary determined, as it has inherent physical limits. Certain paints need a container and are quantity determined: How big is the container holding the liquid? One way to place a medium on the continuum is to determine what kind of container is being used and how the properties need to be contained. Using the finger paints as an example again, note that when an amount is placed on the paper, it stays where it is placed. Not so with tempera paint or inks. Boundaries are either inherent in the materials or made by the participant.

The directives and the distancing agent (brush, hammer, chisel, among others) help serve the purpose of creating boundaries on the use of the media. If several steps are introduced, they must be considered both separately and collectively. The materials need to be able to absorb the use of the mediator appropriately. If a client is given tempera paints and the directive is unstructured, such as "paint anything you wish," then a variety of sizes in brushes and various sizes of paper should be provided. The person can set his or her own boundaries in using the paint. The practitioner is assisting with the resonance of the initiative. However, if the individual is given a small piece of paper and one large brush, then a potentially frustrating experience is created. What is the goal of the initiative? What is being explored about boundaries and emotions? If the brush and the paint are the tools to express the self, is the person too "big" for his or her own personal environment? Does that person "fit" his or her situation? Watch the manner in which this problem is solved or not. An easy directive would be to paint a single self-symbol. A difficult directive would be to create "your world." A good directive would be to "find a way to comfortably express yourself in this space."

Another example of media rich in therapeutic value would be the use of natural clay stoneware. The clay is boundary determined, but its contents may also be considered quantitatively. Thus, the amount of clay given needs to fit the directive and rationale. In some cases, modeling clay is not a good medium, but if it is all that can be afforded choose one of the newer plasticines or self-drying clays. The beauty of clay is its ability to absorb energy and create form from the energy exerted. If the synthetics can do this, use them; however, we recommend the real thing. Get down to earth!

The initiative Clay Haptic-Visual Self (Chapter 5) is a good example of using the media properties to enhance the emotional and cognitive awareness and discover one's own boundaries and/or lack of boundaries in different areas of life.

Symbolic Representation and Interpretation

In this book, we tend toward a Jungian perspective on symbolism but do not deny the role of what Freudian psychoanalysis has called the personal unconscious. In fact, we find that the two may be integrated very well. Most of our clients and students are more aware of a cognitive-based explanation of behavior and the world around them. Since the ETC continuum at the third level starts with the cognitive and yields to the symbolic, this makes sense.

As children, we substitute objects for persons or other objects. This is early symbolism. Later in life, we tend more toward representational thinking until we are confronted with a situation or event that brings up unconscious material and reactions.

Integration of Concepts

These brief exploration of some of the foundations of the ETC can best be understood as integration and continuum of concepts. The table that follows illustrates the relationship among the ETC, graphic development, and Piagetian play development.

Another and very simplistic correlation between the ETC and our understanding of neuroscience may be seen in (1) the Kinesthetic/Sensory relating to the brain-stem (reptilian) functions, (2) the

Table 3.1 Relationship of ETC to Graphic and Play Development

Expressive Therapies Continuum (ETC)	Graphic Development	Play Development
Kinesthetic/Sensory (K/S)	Scribble	Sensorimotor play
Perceptual/Affective (P/A)	Preschematic	Practice play
Cognitive/Symbolic (C/S)	Schematic to Naturalistic	Symbolic play—liquidating-compensatory

Table 3.2 Media Dimension Variables

Media Dimension Variables	
High complexity	Control, problem solving
Low complexity	Allows more emphasis on media properties or symbolic data
Unstructured	Loosening of boundaries; tends to yield more attention to media properties and can enhance creativity
Structured	Boundaries, rules, safety
Fluid	Leans toward the affective
Resistive	Leans toward the cognitive/symbolic but can yield more intense emotions

Perceptual/Affective relating to the limbic system (midbrain), and (3) the Cognitive/Symbolic being the cortical (cortex) functioning. Several authors have elucidated this brilliantly, and we will refer you to Dr. David Siegel and Hass-Cohen (Hass-Cohen and Carr, 2008, and Siegel, 2012). Cathy Malchiodi has also done an excellent job of explaining the trauma-informed practices in expressive therapies to the various brain functions (Malchiodi, 2015). We rejoice that although we have "come of age" in the scientific community, we have not negated the wonder and sometimes mystery of the arts.

References

Hass-Cohen, N. and Carr, N. (Eds.) (2008). *Art Therapy and Clinical Neuroscience*. London: Jessica Kingsley Press.

Huang, T.L. and Charyton, C. (2008). A comprehensive review of the psychological effects of brainwave entrainment. *Alternative Therapies*, Sept/Oct, 14 (5), 38–49.

Kagin, S. (1978). Perception and the encephalopod: Human figure drawings by four year olds. *Art Psychotherapy*, 5, 143–147. Pergamon Press.

Kagin, S. and Lusebrink, V. (1978). The expressive therapies continuum. *Art Psychotherapy*, 5, 171–180. Pergamon Press.

Lowenfeld, V. and Brittain, W.L. (1970). *Creative and Mental Growth* (7th ed.). New York, NY: Macmillan.

Lowenfeld, V. and Brittain, W.L. (1987). *Creative and Mental Growth* (8th ed.). Upper Saddle River, NJ: Prentice Hall.

Malchiodi, C.A. (2015). *Trauma-Informed Expressive Arts Therapy*. New York, NY: Guilford.

Merriam-Webster Dictionary (2015). Springfield, MA: Merriam-Webster.

Piaget, J. (1962). *Play, Dreams and Imitation in Childhood*. New York, NY: Basic Books.

Rhyne, J. (1974). *The Gestalt Art Experience*. Chicago, IL: Magnolia Street Publishers.

Siegel, D. (2012). *Pocket Guide to Interpersonal Neurobiology: An Integrative Handbook of the Mind*. New York, NY: Norton and Company.

CHAPTER 4

Kinesthetic-/Sensory-Focused Initiatives

Introduction to the Clinical Practice Guide

At the Kinesthetic/Sensory (K/S) level, the sensorimotor stage of cognitive development (Piaget, 1969) is translated into behavior both elicited from and enhanced by the media properties. It can be very important therapeutically to be two years old expressively, even if one is 20, 30, or 40 chronologically. The purpose is to experience pure sensory input that forms and leads to emotional awareness and the development of memory.

At an even more simplistic level, the K/S initiatives activate brain stem (reptilian brain) synaptic discharge:

- Activates awareness of basic bodily functions
- Stimulates reticular activating system wakefulness
- Initiates fight, flight, or freeze response
- Connects states of energy and information flow
- Enhances self-compassion
- Breaks free from cortical control

The following pages include initiatives that serve as examples of kinesthetic and sensory experiences. As in all the initiatives in this guide, we have written the directives as if we were speaking to the client or student, giving the reader a script to follow.

Initiative One—Scribble Chase Mural

ETC—Kinesthetic/Sensory (K/S), Perceptual/Affective (P/A), Cognitive/Symbolic (C/S)

MDV—High Complexity Unstructured Fluid (HCUF)

One of the most basic experiences we use in art therapy is scribble drawing. It originally was a template by which unconscious materials were manifested and form was found that had symbolic meaning. We have expanded on this in the first of our initiatives.

Materials

Washable markers, newsprint (12 × 18), or white butcher paper

Directives

1. Divide into pairs. Each pair will choose a sheet of newsprint and a set of markers for the scribble chase. Using only eye contact, one of you will begin the scribble while the other follows. Switch roles midway through the process. Do not discuss who will lead or follow verbally but by body language and connection with each other.
2. Find at least five images or objects within the scribbles and agree on the five to be taken to the next grouping. Obviously, these may be discussed.
3. Each pair should now groups with another pair to form a group of four persons. As a new group, decide upon five images from the original composite of 10.
4. Combine with another group of four, making eight persons to decide which five images from the two groups will be selected with which to make a mural.
5. Using markers and referring to the five images chosen, draw a group mural. The actual images need not be used, but the ideas of the images may be created on the mural.
6. Note your own thoughts, feelings, and behaviors at each level of functioning from the original pair to a group of eight. Write these down under "Personal Comments."

Rationale—Great Introduction to All the Levels of the ETC

When two people face each other over a blank piece of paper and are directed to "chase" each other, they will engage in behaviors that provide insight into how they react to someone without words, toning the other senses, as well as whether such interaction arouses anxiety, curiosity, confusion, or frustration. This is a very good project to use with a couple in a relationship or within members of a family or as an icebreaker in a new group. Its use in therapy, educational settings, and team leadership training, for example, gives a picture of who in a group commands dominance, who is more submissive, who rebels, or who is simply playful.

It is often difficult for an individual to be the "leader" or the "follower," and since the experience is largely *kinesthetic*, it also taps into inhibition and boundary challenges, as well as aggression or passivity. The scribble behavior is that of a very young child. Look for and ask about regression. The markers are a *fluid* medium and should assist a "flow" as one resonates with the material.

Below are some guidelines and question prompts a therapist might provide during this activity:

Did the experience feel "silly" or "freeing"? Does the behavior fit a pattern of other behaviors in your life? Processing can lead them to recall childhood experiences, and they can be encouraged to discuss them.

Look at the use of the paper as a metaphorical life space and see how much is used, how expansive or constricted the lines are, what colors were chosen, and how much pressure was used. Compare being the leader with being the follower. Which is more comfortable? This is an introduction to learning one's visual language as well as learning about projection and the unconscious as it is exhibited on the paper.

How easy or difficult was it for the pairs to find images in the scribbles? Moving from the kinesthetic and perceptual (form) levels to the cognitive/symbolic (naming the forms) can be a challenge for some people who are concrete thinkers.

How did the two people go about choosing and agreeing on five images? Do these images have any personal meaning? Were there one or two images that one of the pair simply had to have on the image selection? What were these images? Changing to a new group allows the participant to test resiliency and adaptability. Did the participant's behavior change with a group of four then a group of eight? What kind of negotiation strategies were used to decide on the images? Did the leadership change? Did the thoughts and feelings of each participant change? Is this also a life pattern? Is the individual comfortable with it, or does he or she wish to make changes? All of these thoughts will be written in the "Personal Comments" for students or in a journal for clients or simply discussed verbally in processing.

After the group completes its project, the group dynamics and contribution of each member become the focus. Does the mural have a theme?

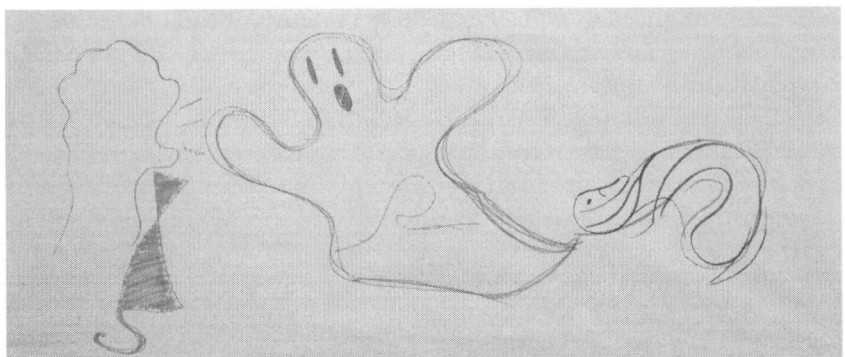

Figure 4.1 Scribble Chase Mural

Did the group work well together and equally? Who decided to draw what? These are all questions for the group upon completion of their art.

A great amount of information may be derived from the final product. The processing is limited only by the time in session. However, a picture is taken of the mural at the end of the session for later feedback and reflection.

Figure 4.1 shows a mural on white butcher paper with a ghost, a cat, and a sideways swan.

Personal Comments—21-Year-Old Female Undergraduate Student of Professor Kagin

We each made one continuous line. I felt more comfortable leading. I think our group had the most trouble finding shapes and I pressed very hard. We took turns finding images/didn't see the same things but did once the other person showed us. The group was interesting. No one really communicated. It was kind of like we were walking on eggshells and not connected, like our objects. I felt like I could have steam rolled the project but held back because I was trying to see other people's perspectives and not taking charge as I sort of did with my partner. I had to watch myself.

Therapeutic Transition

Looking back at the mural in Figure 4.1, it is important to note that this exercise came at the beginning of the class. Two other initiatives had preceded this, both of which were individual projects. In processing, students recognized that this mural shows an uncertainty about group dynamics and each person's role. It also visually communicates a lack of communication between the participants. While each person added marks to the paper, there was no discussion to support those marks.

It might be of interest that according to Jung, the ghost (as seen in the mural) represents consciousness without a brain or unconscious complexes undergoing change, conflict, or integration (Ronnberg and Martin, 2010). It would be enlightening for the group to discuss their "ghost" and how each contributes to keeping it alive and powerful as the largest image on the paper.

Our commentator reported holding herself back and the experience of walking on eggshells. She expressed fear in these statements and was clearly reticent in her actions. Encouraging her but also the group to engage in verbal communication would safely give her opportunities to feel out the situations prior to engaging and thus would help her to not regress and hold back. It is clear that this group needed more specific directives, because due to the small size of the group, Directives 3 and 4 were not possible, which limited communication.

Creativity Activation

The creativity level is achieved at several phases, including the process of idea generation, which comes from the fluency of the scribble chase and the originality in finding forms from the ambiguous lines; story conception, when the group works together with images to formulate the story (motivation, producing, sharing); and the point of image creation, when the mural takes form (implementing). Integration of the various levels of the ETC and MDV produces the catalyst for the creativity as clients work with materials and one another.

Adaptations

The scribble chase could be used again at a midpoint in therapy to open the client up to a free association and compare responses to the art processes from the beginning of therapy to those in the present. It could also be used at a midpoint for a group to explore group dynamics and progress. More specific directives or questions, such as "How do these symbols (shapes) work together or how would you want them to work together?" or "How will you decide the placement and scale of your objects?" could initiate communication if the family or group is small and can only pair once and then move to the larger group. Educationally, this could also initiate a discussion of how families differ and how to accept these differences.

The scribbling portion could be introduced in one group and images could be identified and discussed, with the actual mural being produced in the next session. This facilitates more time to reflect on the story and return for cohesion. Paint or other media may be used to aid expression of feelings. Movement exercises may be used before starting to begin the free-flowing, sweeping arm movements. The Scribble Chase Mural can be used as an individual project to allow one person to explore scribbling and finding images. For those experiencing anxiety with the art process, therapists could use a smaller piece of paper. For clients with attention-deficit/hyperactivity disorder (ADHD), this could be used as a focusing exercise, one that could be done on their own outside of therapy.

Initiative Two—Expressions in Movement and Sound

ETC—all, especially Kinesthetic/Sensory (K/S)
MDV—High Complexity Unstructured Resistive (HCUR)

The experiences introduced with this initiative give the clinician and participant a taste of the intermodal functioning at the Kinesthetic/Sensory and Perceptual level. The end result becomes Cognitive/Symbolic. The regressive nature of the scribble and vocal connection is or can be especially powerful, as the limbic system may awaken memories starting at around age 2 (early Scribble Stage) and sensorimotor repetitive play. This is a group project and requires a fairly large room with empty space for moving.

Materials

Large crayons, newsprint (12 × 18) or large sheet of butcher (mural) paper, assorted percussion instruments (enough for each participant to use at least one). If budget is an issue or actual instruments are unavailable, then cans and sticks and sandpaper, bells, wooden or metal spoons, or similar items may be substituted.

Directives

1. Sit on the floor and pretend to be two years old again. Draw and scribble on the paper. While scribbling, make sounds that go with the actions or lines of the scribble. Make two or three scribble pages.
2. Begin to be more aware of the sounds your group is making and less aware of the scribbles. (By virtue of entrainment, a group chant will evolve after a short period of time.)
3. Choose one of your own drawings and find an instrument that makes a sound that you think expresses the drawing.
4. Assemble, standing in a circle, with the drawing at your feet, and use your instrument to illustrate your drawing. Go around the circle one by one to be sure each person participates.
5. Staying in the circle, go around again and ask each participant to make a movement to express the drawing. Now simultaneously everyone in the group should make a movement, vocal sound, and instrument sound all at once.

Continue until a rhythm spontaneously evolves in both movement and sound.
6. Have someone volunteer to be the "conductor" of the group. This person will then align the group and choreograph a group dance using movement and sound. Once the group has begun, the conductor will step back into the group and an ending will naturally evolve.
7. Process as a group, and each participant will individually write down their reactions as well. Focus on trying to be two years old again. How did that feel, and did any feelings emerge as you were scribbling? Was your scribbling loose or tight, controlled or spontaneous? Did your reaction change by the third drawing and if so, how? How easy or difficult was it to make sounds as you scribbled? How would you describe your sound? Did any feelings evolve from just making sound with your movements?
8. When you became aware of the sounds the group was making, which captured your attention first? Did you find yourself adapting to that sound? How long did it take for a chant to evolve and why?
9. How easy or difficult was it to transfer your drawing to an instrument? What instrument did you choose? Were you satisfied with your translation of your scribble?
10. Were you comfortable demonstrating your drawing and instrument rendition? Did any one particular person capture your attention more than others in their presentation? Why?
11. Who was the conductor, and how was the conductor chosen? Did you like the way the performance was conducted? Did you prefer leadership or being on your own with the group when the conductor rejoined you?
12. Overall, what did you learn about yourself throughout this initiative? What did you learn about the ETC and MDV?

See Figure 4.2 by a 35-year-old mental health professional from a group led by Dr. Graves-Alcorn. In this image, the drawing includes layers of mark making with various media. The directional lines move spontaneously across the ground and even have dots and C-shaped marks placed within and over curvilinear lines and sharp jagged blue lines.

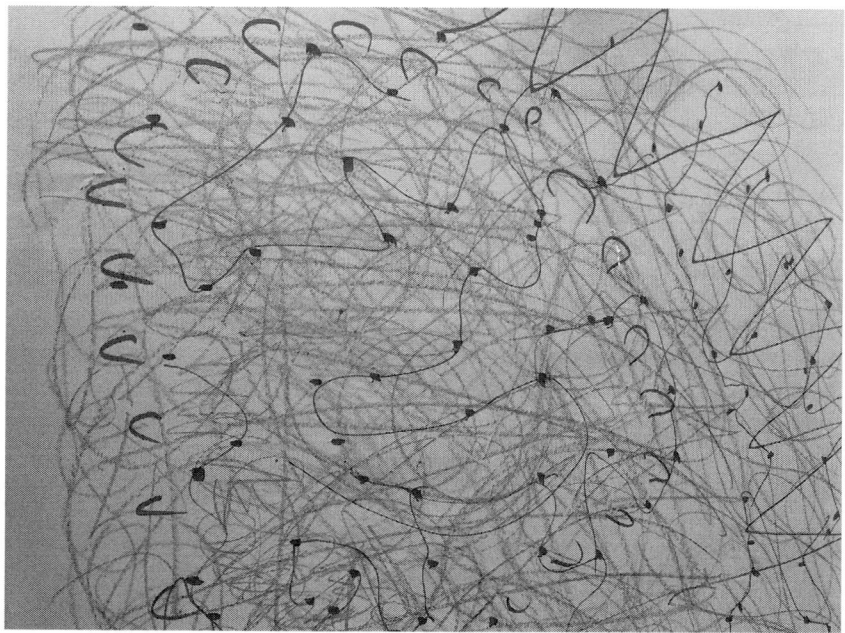

Figure 4.2 Expressions in Movement and Sound

Personal Comments—35-Year-Old Mental Health Professional from a Group Led by Dr. Graves-Alcorn

It was hard to imagine being a two year old. I know not to make complete shapes or figures but had to consciously stop myself. Crayons are a more natural choice for a two year old. I was not interested in making any kind of noise/sound with my mouth. I wanted to make noise with the crayon—banging with the crayon. Making noise with the instrument was also intimidating but I appreciated using the ridge sticks. The stamping also seemed similar to noise with the crayons. The group music and movement felt more integrated. I appreciated the different levels.

Therapeutic Transition

This participant noted in her personal comments at least two areas of strength on which further initiatives could follow, creating form and problem solving. She got bored when she was not doing something more complex and putting ideas together. When we think of bored, what feeling emerges? She mentioned having difficulty being a 2-year-old. We would ask why and wonder if she is more wired for high-arousal challenges. At the same time she does not respond well to authoritative people, refusing to make the sounds with her mouth, so a less structured approach may be best. Depending upon her therapeutic goals, the next step may be High Complexity Unstructured Resistive (HCUR). She probably flourishes on being in charge with plenty of stimulation and options open to her. It will be helpful for her to consider how she feels and reacts when she is not in charge and whether this has caused her any problems. Since regression is an issue, it may be difficult for her to "play" and loosen the boundaries she either creates or in which she finds herself. If we were to speculate that the "banging" with the crayons that created dots represented parts of her, challenges, issues, or control points, it would be good to have her "connect the dots" and create a form then free associate to that form.

Creativity Activation

The creativity level is achieved first when divergent thinking is necessary when the instrument is selected as applicable to the visual and played to express the drawing in Directive 3. The kinesthetic is connected to the sensory, and idea generation is initiated. The next full activation of the creativity level is achieved in Directive 6, when the group together finds a rhythm and works together (producing, sharing, and implementing). This process elicits from the participant both an intrinsic and an extrinsic motivation response that aligns to others. Finding a unification of the sounds and movements and participating therein is building on previous information and dedication to problem solving, which results in creative engagement.

Adaptations

The dynamics of the group's interaction may be emphasized. Pairs could work together to create movement and sound for each other and then give feedback. The visuals could be lined up according to group decision and the movement/sound be more structured by the sequence of the visuals. A related directive may be to make the instruments using scrap supplies gathered by the group. This activity would also spark creative problem solving.

For groups with difficulty in body awareness, the facilitator could begin with stretching or other movement exercise to help them become more comfortable. If issues of respecting others' space arise or are expected, each person could be assigned to a specific area marked by hula hoops or tape squares on the floor. Allow those insecure with their movement or sound to pass on the individual display but to participate in the group display.

Choreographing the group into a unified dance by asking each person to demonstrate the chosen movement and sound then following with the entire group mimicking those movements creates a powerful adaptation for group cohesion. After the first demonstration, the group would mimic each movement and play the sounds. By the end, the entire group would participate in one fluid dance to which each member contributed.

Initiative Three—Media Properties and Range of Materials

ETC—Kinesthetic/Sensory (K/S)
MDV—Low Complexity Unstructured Fluid and Resistive (LCUFR)

This initiative may be used in a classroom, in an art therapy group, or as a client assessment tool.

The significance of this initiative is slightly different than other initiatives because it is also a critical element of learning for the art therapy student. While a client's exploration of media for assessment is the foundational substance of this initiative, it has been used to educate future art therapists as to their own responses and experiences with materials but also to deepen their understanding of the clients' experience to better equip them with knowledge, empathy, and direction. In a classroom context, students are expected to use all of the media in this exercise, not to make choices. This is essential, because one must know and investigate the properties of a material and one's personal responses to its manipulation for therapeutic application. If a client is given a material with which to work with a specific directive because the goal is to facilitate the concentration on an issue or emotion, the therapist must be fully aware of its properties and must also be able to understand how a positive or a negative response to a material impacts the outcome and emotion of a client. Therefore, an adaptation of this initiative is for art therapy students to use all materials and rate them on a Likert scale (Likert, 1932) with personal comments.

Materials

It is essential that a large room with several tables be available. Each table may be set up for one or two experiences, giving enough room for at least two people at each station. The focus is on the material properties. There is no direction for use, so complexity and structure are minimized and depend on the individual response. If this experience is contained within a certain time limit, then establish the amount of time to be spent at each station. For example, in our lab, we had an hour and a half, and each student was given 10 minutes per station. If it is possible to do this in two sessions or even more, the assessment value increases without the time stressor.

PAPERS—small and large drawing paper (8½ × 11 and 12 × 18), large pieces of newsprint, colored construction paper (8½ × 11), colored art tissue (these come in large sheets), finger paint paper (12 × 18), watercolor paper (sketchbook size), and canvas board

PAINTS—finger paints, watercolor in tubes and in blocks, tempera paint, acrylics in tubes. Since oils involve more than just the paint, we have left these out. Be certain that at least the primary colors plus black and white are available. Also have trays for mixing and bowls of water next to the paints.

DRAWING MATERIALS—pencils with eraser (No. 2), colored pencils, markers, large and small crayons, oil pastels, regular pastels, graphite sticks

3-D—natural clay, plasticine, modeling clay, wood scraps, wood squares or rectangles for backgrounds, metal scraps, ceramic tiles, clay tools, hammer and various nails, glue (Elmer's and E-6,000), pieces of cloth for cleanup, and water bowls

MIXED MEDIA—string, straws, inks, yarn, variety of pieces of different-textured cloth materials, cotton balls, polymer liquid, scraps of wallpaper and foils, beads of different sizes, feathers, sparkle confetti or sparkle glue, scissors, poster board, textured objects for printing, including sponges and print designs, ink pads

Any other materials you can afford or imagine plus lots of cleanup supplies!

It is important to inquire whether the person has used any of the materials presented before. If he or she is experienced in a medium, be sure that is noted on the scale provided, as it may bias the response.

Directives

1. Look around the room and see the variety of materials available to you. (Therapist identifies materials for those who may not be familiar with them.)
2. Each person will use the materials in whatever way desired, but each material needs to be used individually, not together, except for the mixed media.
3. Once you have used the material, give a rating scale for each project. The following is an example, but you may create your own. The one below is created on a Likert scale of 1 to 7 (see Box 4.1).

The art does the work for you! After the individual has experienced and rated each material(s), it is very informative to lay out the rating scales and find commonalities.

```
MEDIUM (Name of Material)
PROPERTY (Fluid to Resistive)
  1     2     3     4     5     6     7
REINFORCEMENT VALUE (Dislike to Like)
  1     2     3     4     5     6     7
PERSONAL ENERGY (Low to High Arousal)
  1     2     3     4     5     6     7
```

Box 4.1 Rating Scale for MDV Lab

Personal Comments

For example, one student used the tissue paper and glue to create "flowers." She "crushed" the tissue onto construction paper and glued it. She also added some flowered fabric for a border. She rated this a 3 between fluid and resistive, a 1 for Reinforcement value, and 1 for Personal energy. She had a similar rating for cray-pas and pastels; however, the tempera and finger paint were high in the personal energy and reinforcement values, rating them as 4s and 5s. What might this mean to her? When she created her own High Complexity Resistive project, she did not like it. However, when she resonated with the more fluid materials, her reinforcement value went up.

If you are working with her, where would you lead her? Where would she lead herself? Ask!

Therapeutic Transition

We advise that in most cases, you begin with experiences most comfortable to the client. This lady obviously prefers the more fluid materials and less complexity in directives. Give her choices of paints, sizes of brushes, and paper. Directives should guide toward the affective range.

Creativity Activation

As clients work with the various media, incubation is activated first in the kinesthetic problem solving of what to do with the materials and, second, intrinsic motivation is activated if resonating has occurred. If no illumination results, then the reinforcement value of the production will be rated low. This gives insight or produces curiosity as to why one or more of the properties "fit" with the individual's personality.

Adaptation

This initiative can take place over a period of time, through multiple sessions, rather than in the sequence we developed. If it is divided by media and each grouping is introduced one at a time, it has the ability to provide the clients with a historical review of their emotional and sensory responses and keep record of their progress.

Initiative Four—Visual Breathing

ETC—Kinesthetic/Sensory (K/S)
MDV—Low Complexity Unstructured Fluid (LCUF)

This initiative has a multitude of uses. It can be used in the classroom for focus with adolescents or teens, or it could be used with grade school children for calming and recognition of energy. It has been used at the start and end of art therapy sessions, in the clinical methods courses for art therapy students, and in journals of students and clients. It is a good ongoing practice for overall insight and focus and fostering the beginning of flow (which is discussed in Chapter 7 on creativity).

Over time, continued use of this initiative in a journal provides an opportunity for individuals to learn their visual language (patterns of marks, line quality variations, and color changes at various times in their day-to-day life) and distinguish various moods, both during times of stress and in times of calm. Becoming aware of breathing changes and similarities by exploring them visually can help make connections between situations clients might not see interrelated otherwise.

Materials

18 × 24 drawing paper, markers or pastels

Directives

1. Begin by getting comfortable. Settle into your seat. Relax your arms into your lap or onto the table. Relax your shoulders. Put your feet flat on the floor.
2. Close your eyes.
3. Take a deep breath into your body and slowly release it.
4. Breathe in again, slow and deep. As your breath moves into your body, notice how your body moves with the breath.
5. With slow, deep breaths, begin to fully feel how your breath is moving through your body.
6. Now visualize your breath as it moves. What color is it? Is it more than one color?
7. With the color in mind, and still taking slow, deep breaths, see your breath moving through your body. Is it rapid or slow movement? Does it move faster coming in than it does going out? Or does it come in slowly and go out quickly? Is the

movement consistent? Does it flow smoothly? Try to see and feel your breath. Have the colors changed? Is there only one?
8. Once you have become fully aware of your breath, its colors, and movement, focus on this and then open your eyes.
9. With markers or pastels, draw your breath as you saw it and felt it.
10. Process.

Rationale

Mindfulness is actively becoming aware. This breathing exercise that takes the meditative act of slow and deep breathing and transforms it into a visual representation engages the client in body awareness. Nonthreatening, this awareness centers and focuses the client's thoughts on color and movement, not body form or the suppression of thoughts. The body and mind can relax as the visual color moves into and out of the body. The act of drawing the movement with color provides an external expression of calm.

This directive can be used before the start of each session.

In Figures 4.3 and 4.4, by a 20-year-old female student of Professor Kagin, there is consistency in the marks and a similarity in the

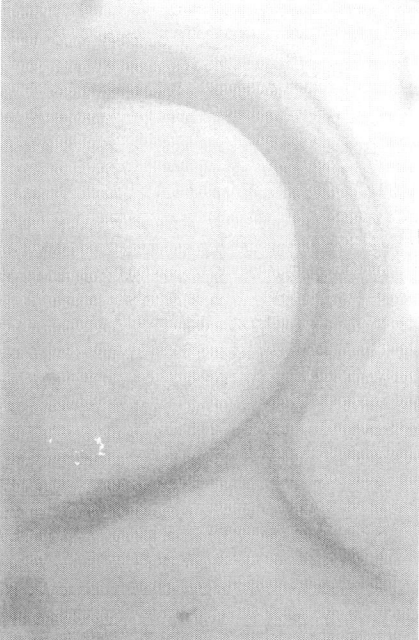

Figure 4.3 Visual Breathing

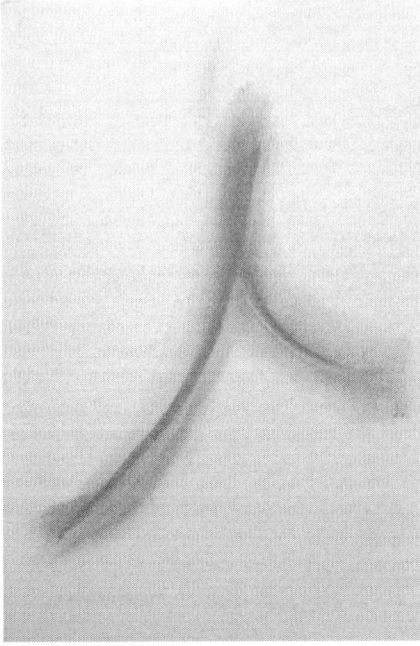

Figure 4.4 Visual Breathing

movement of the stroke of the pastel. While there is a color change, the woman can see the inward and upward movement of the breath and the downward and out exhale. Noticing how while one is more curved and full and the other is more vertical, yet the movement has consistency, can be informative for her, leading her to ask questions, such as, what significance does the color variation have to how she was feeling at the time? How does the crescent shaped breath vary from the more vertical breath in relationship to mood, physical status, or stress?

This can be further explored as a correlation to the much larger drawing in Figure 4.5 (18 × 24 pastel Visual Breathing at beginning of group session), which shows a visual breathing exercise led by the words, "Get comfortable in your chair, focus on your breath. Begin to inhale slowly, and exhale. As you do, become aware of the colors and movement of your breath as it enters in and exits out. When you have a full visual, begin to draw." In this drawing, there is still a vertical movement, though more shallow, and the visual breath has layers of color (blue, green, violet) that are heavier and more grounded at the bottom and soften to a haze at the top. There is a similar movement

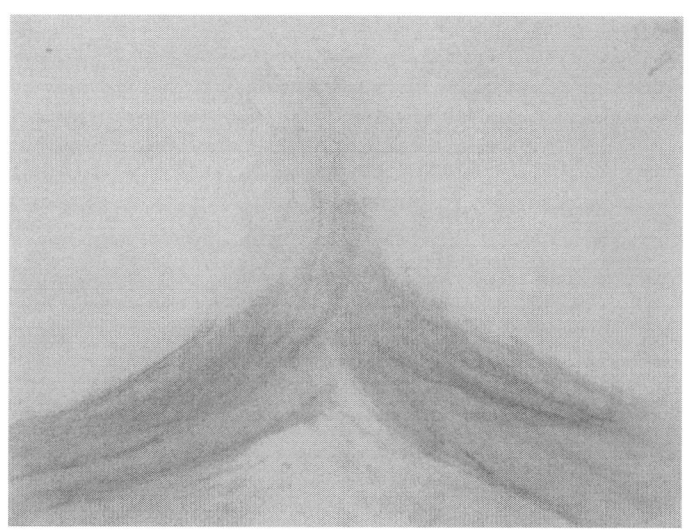

Figure 4.5 Visual Breathing

of the hand and stroke of the pastel, but this time more colors and repetitive lines have been used.

For the student, it is good to note that the two journal entries were completed at times chosen by her as part of the homework to record visual breathing in a journal at various times through the week, while the second was completed at the start of class. Her personal comments that follow speak to her experience with visual breathing overall, not just the three examples here.

Personal Comments—21-Year-Old Undergraduate Student of Professor Kagin

Student One

It feels very grounding. It allows me to be still, be totally present to the moment as I am all focused on how it feels and the color of my breath. My strokes are almost always the same to represent my breath, but the color varies a lot. The stroke is how it feels moving through my body while the color is more how I feel emotionally. The breath always feels like it comes to a peak through me when I inhale and then calmly flows out when I exhale.

In Figures 4.6 and 4.7, by a 20-year-old undergraduate student of Professor Kagin, the Visual Breathing marks are strongly contrasted to Figures 4.3, 4.4, and 4.5. These drawings have visible layers of very

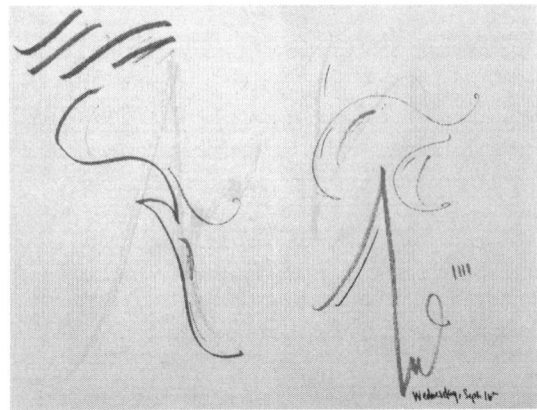

Figure 4.6 Visual Breathing

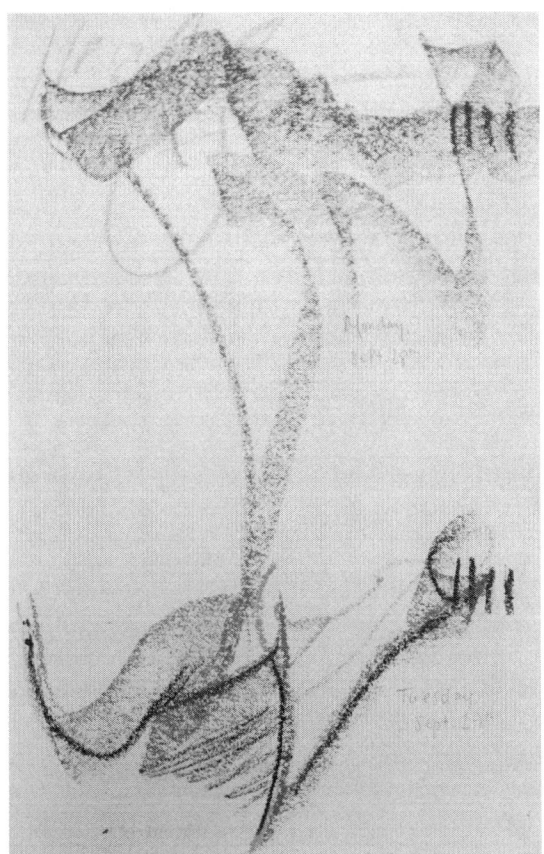

Figure 4.7 Visual Breathing

distinct colors and marks that overlap and also exist on their own. In both Figures 4.6 and 4.7, there is a strong vertical movement with a harsh point and a release that moves downward, followed by another movement upward, though more shallow. The color varies and the medium varies but again, consistency and pattern can be seen.

Personal Comments — 20-Year-Old Undergraduate Student

Student Two
Visual Breathing, for me, was something that held great weight. Although it was assigned for class most times, it was something that gave me the opportunity to stop for a moment and really take a step back. To look at my day, or experience in front of me with an expectancy to change me was what this exercise did for me. It allowed me to look at the miniscule moments throughout the day and see how they fit in to where I ended up at the end of the night. To look through my journal a few months in and see the overall consistency in line quality and then have some that were completely different was very striking. It was a reminder of the part of me that is consistent throughout life, and yet the outside influences that are so prevalent in any part of life.

Therapeutic Transition

The students' experiences as shown in the marked differences between Student One and Student Two indicated that the second young woman appeared to be more anxious and less relaxed. The initiative that could follow would be to ask her to draw her mood states—mad, sad, glad, and scared—and compare them to the image of her visual breathing. Student One appears ready to move on to any initiative directed, as she appears open and willing.

Creativity Activation

The imagination is actively engaged in the visualization of breathing through fluency and originality of creating marks on the page. This change of focus from simply being aware of the breath to giving it color and movement activates a problem-solving response to a life function and becomes intrinsically motivating through repetition.

Adaptations

This directive can be used at the start of group sessions to bring everyone together in a single act and focus them. It can also be used at the start of individual sessions. Clients can be asked to keep a journal of visual breathing to help them become more fully aware of the colors and marks they make during different emotional states. Completing visual breathing in times of stress or anxiety or even anger allows the person to become aware of how these emotions impact their breathing. It may also help them be more aware of their heartbeat.

This exercise is given to students as part of their journaling practice to inform them of patterns and color preference related to mood and to make them aware of mark-making changes. This regular act becomes meditative and serves as a mindfulness act for self-awareness.

References

Likert, R. (1932). A technique for the measurement of attitudes. *Archives of Psychology*, 140, 1–55.

Piaget, J. (1969). *The Psychology of the Child*. New York, NY: Basic Books.

Ronnberg, A. (Ed. in chief) and Martin, K. (Ed.) (2010). *The Book of Symbols: Reflections on Archetypal Images*. Cologne, Germany: Taschen.

CHAPTER 5
Perceptual-/Affective-Focused Initiatives

The Perceptual/Affective level is the continuation of the K/S experiences focusing on emotional awareness and activates the limbic region of the brain. This brain activity:

Helps process autobiographical and explicit factual memory
Perceives and mediates emotional responses, especially fear and anger
Controls impact of hormones and the stress cycle.

Initiative Five—Expressive Drawings: Mind States—Mood States

ETC—Kinesthetic/Sensory (K/S) and Perceptual/Affective (P/A)
MDV—High Complexity Structured Fluid (HCSF)

Much of this material was developed while Dr. Janie Rhyne was on the faculty at the University of Louisville. Already known for her work in Gestalt art therapy (Rhyne, 1974), she was fascinated by visual constructs and spent much time studying the work of Rudolph Arnheim, David Dondis, and George Kelley. She was particularly interested in balance that involves constructs of horizontal versus vertical orientation, with diagonal or oblique orientations seeming to threaten equilibrium in a work of art (Agell, 1998). She was also fascinated by polarities such as regularity versus simplicity, orderly versus chaotic, harmony versus discord, and ambiguity versus clarity. Dondis (1973) articulated the visual elements of the dot, the line, and shape. Rhyne broke these down into representational form, symbolic form, and abstract form. She noted that "the specific problem addressed . . . is the examination of how form relationships convey meaning in their structural dimensions of compositional organization" (Rhyne, 1979).

Rhyne further delineated the structural properties she was studying: visual dynamics of form relationships, orientations, directed movement, spatial interactions, and kinesthetic qualities. The movements in the drawing (upward or downward), pushing outward or pulling inward, dominating space or opening to the space, closing, around the edges, heaviness pulling downward, bursts of upward movement, all were found to be of significance when paired with a stimulus word such as "depression," "guilt," "going crazy," "being sane," "serene," "anxious," "angry," and other emotional descriptors.

It is unfortunate that Rhyne never published this dissertation, as it was a seminal work. Her findings have been used by Graves-Alcorn and others in courtroom testimony regarding the emotional states of persons of interest.

One of the most basic objectives of art therapy is to teach the participant their own visual language as well as to assist in the translation of a feeling into visual form. This initiative helps to develop a visual "dictionary" as well as translate the emotions "mad," "sad," "glad," and "scared" into color and form. Other mind states than those listed here may be used.

Materials

Colored markers, 13 sheets of 8 ½ × 11 white paper, 4 sheets of 12 × 18 watercolor paper, full range of tempera or acrylic paints, several sizes of brushes, bowls of water

Directives

1. Drawing quickly and spontaneously, listen to each word as I say it and draw your response to it using only line, form, and color; illustrate each directive. Each word, or mind state, will be on a separate piece of paper. Do not use symbols or representations such as smiley faces, frowns, question marks, or any other more objective response. These need to be abstractions of your perception of the word given.
2. When you have finished drawing, turn the page over and use your pencil to indicate which mind state you have just drawn.
3. The mind-state words are as follows:
   Anxious
   Fearful
   Going crazy
   Hoping
   Depressed
   Being sane
   Threatened
   Guilty
   Joyous
   Passive
   Hostile
   Serene
   Compassionate
4. When all 13 have been completed, put them aside and do not refer to them until directed to do so.
5. Using the large sheets of paper and the paint, express these four mood states, each on a separate piece of paper. Paint in whatever order chosen.
   Mad
   Sad
   Glad
   Scared
6. Spread the 13 mind states out and arrange them according to similarities in salient features of the abstract drawing

(placement, form, line, direction, filling space, and other visual elements).
7. Next, lay out the four mood-state paintings.
8. Match the groupings of salient features of mind states with those of the mood states. Lay them out so there is enough space to observe the work.
9. Write down the results (which mind states were clustered with which mood states).

Rationale

Each individual has a personal set of visual constructs, but as Scheerer and Lyons (1957) have shown, there is also a universal quality to these constructs in design, shape, patterning, dominant direction, pressure, and closure in line drawings and matching responses to words.

Rhyne's dissertation research contributes to an individual's ability to learn his or her own visual language. The assumption that visual representations of states of mind are experienced by all normal adults gives us the opportunity to develop an expressive visual dictionary, which we can learn to "read" and from which we gain insight, perspective, and creative enrichment (Rhyne, 1979).

For assessment purposes, we may discover deviations from the norms that become helpful in diagnosis and treatment. Here we are comparing and correlating the most basic of emotions as they relate to other experiences in our lives.

As therapists, our greatest challenge is to help our clients and students sort out and clarify these functional emotional patterns and how they are used in daily living in order to gain more resiliency. More often than not, our clients have a "cluttered" perception of feelings, which become overwhelming. Helping to sort out anger from sadness and fear and determine which is the most accessible and used for that individual can be life changing.

Figures 5.1, 5.2, 5.3, and 5.4 were completed by an undergraduate student in her 20s who was in Professor Kagin's class. These are images of Mad (Figure 5.1), Sad (Figure 5.2), Scared (Figure 5.3), and Glad (Figure 5.4).

Personal Comments—20-Year-Old Female Undergraduate Student of Professor Kagin

This exercise really pushed me to think of different visuals that actually represented the mood/mind states. It's one thing to be given four words to visualize, but sixteen really pushes you to come up with things and put thought into

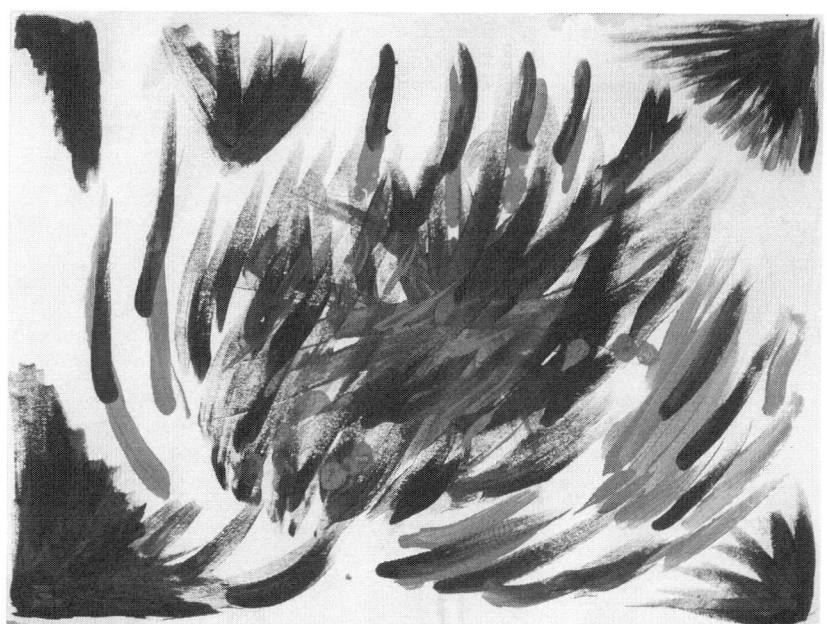

Figure 5.1 Expressive Drawings: Mind States—Mood States (Mad)

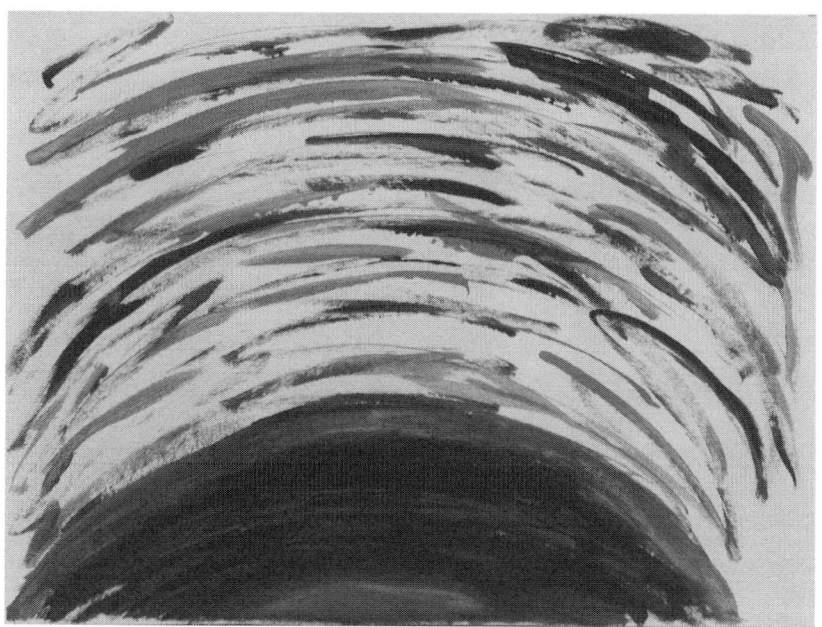

Figure 5.2 Expressive Drawings: Mind States—Mood States (Sad)

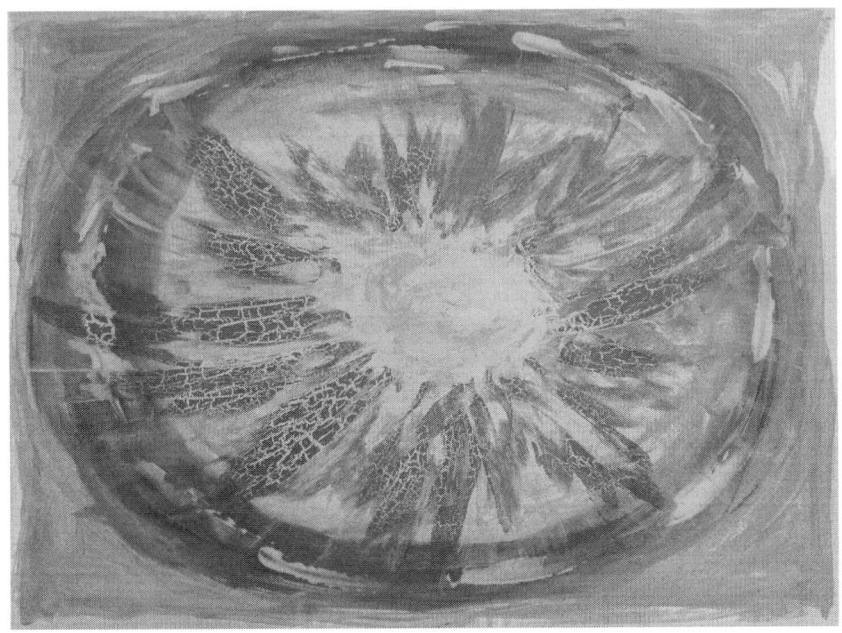

Figure 5.3 Expressive Drawings: Mind States—Mood States (Glad)

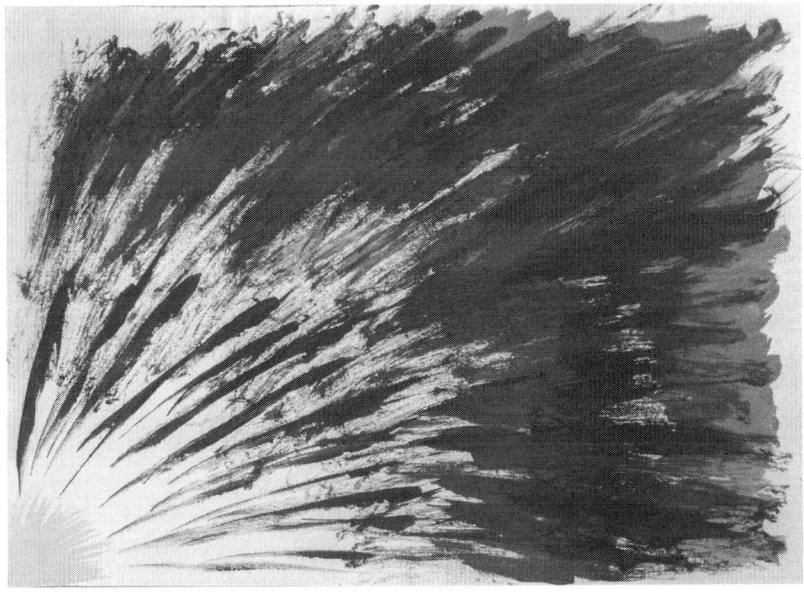

Figure 5.4 Expressive Drawings: Mind States—Mood States (Scared)

it. The high number was essential to having this be a successful exercise. It was very cool flipping the papers over eventually to see what the states were and how they were grouped.

All the words that were together had certain similarities in the way that I would react in situations that I would feel the words describe and other words that correlate, such as guilt and sadness and compassion; almost always we feel guilty because we have made someone sad, and we care about hurting because of the compassion we contain.

Group One words are glad, joyous, going crazy, being sane and hostile. All these words hold a lot of energy that can be suppressed in certain situations. Although they are different words, a lot of them can be assigned the same sort of reaction, simply an output of energy/emotion.

Group Two words are sad, guilty, compassionate. These three words all usually have to do with other people. I find it interesting that they all had similar visuals, "radiate" is a word I use to describe the visual which is a good word to describe one emotion that is associated with not just the person experiencing the particular emotion.

Group Three words are sad, depressed, serene, passive. These four words make me think of extremely inactive behavior, keeping to oneself mostly, and the visuals all do not have very much movement or energy contained within the marks.

Group Four words are scared, hoping, threatened, fearful, anxious. This group of words all look to the future it seems. They make me think of anticipation. When one looks at the visuals they are pretty sporadic marks, and when anticipating something, one usually has a hard time focusing and is not at ease. That feeling is very present in these visuals it seems.

Therapeutic Transition

This young lady has used visuals that fit beautifully into Rhyne's universal language. Since they are well attuned to the emotion expressed, we can assume that she is not suppressing or exaggerating her feelings and is fairly comfortable with them. Her success with this initiative leads us to continue with other perceptual affective experiences, as she seems to gain quite a bit of information from them. Additionally, however, the image of scared looks very threatening. It would be interesting for her to explore areas within the self that may feel uncomfortable and take her via guided imagery to the meadow and the source at the cognitive/symbolic level.

Creativity Activation

Simplifying mood states and mind states into line and color and completing the drawing and painting into one 50-minute session requires the client to express an emotion with swift marks and spontaneous color choices. This type of exercise often leads to enhanced tolerance for ambiguity and problem solving by lessening the cognitive influence. Illumination may occur when the divergent thinking of pairing the images is required. The individual now has new information to use in the future and has begun to develop an emotional dictionary for use in problem solving and greater insight.

Adaptation

While adaptations can include changing the word choices for the mood states and mind states, and perhaps clients could complete the drawings in one session and map them in another and then process, we feel it is best to stay true to Rhyne's procedures. Nonetheless, this exercise has been used in drawing classes with mind states only in which students are exploring the qualities of line and the expressiveness of drawing emotions. In these instances, mood states are not painted, and processing and mapping are not used. The exercise's focus is on the expressive freedom of making marks to communicate an emotion and then discussing the variations within the class. Adaptations and similarities are explored to teach about the communicative language of line.

Initiative Six—Dyadic Nonverbal Communication

ETC—Focus on Perceptual/Affective (P/A) but also Kinesthetic/ Sensory (K/S) and Cognitive (C)
MDV—Low Complexity Unstructured Fluid (LCUF)

The function of nonverbal communication for the therapeutic setting is to allow clients the opportunity to explore the mode of drawing, becoming increasingly aware of their own feelings as they "dialogue" visually with another and as they assert or withdraw from engagement. This initiative requires that a participant interact with multiple people in nonverbal dialogue. Images as well as body language will be the communicators.

Materials

Colored markers, three sheets of 12 × 18 paper

Directives

1. Find a partner and draw using only line and form. All communication should be nonverbal and avoid using symbols such as smiley faces or stick figures. Take 10 minutes to complete. Verbally process the interaction and drawing between the two of you.
2. Repeat this exercise two more times, each time with a different partner.
3. In a small group, take turns as pairs to tell the group what happened during the experience. Discuss how you felt when your partner communicated different ways using line, color, form, and body language. Be aware of any emotions that resulted during the communication.
4. Explore the metaphors evoked by this initiative and what they tell you. Entering the transference/countertransference arena can happen very quickly. Use with care and know your own boundaries and triggers before you proceed.

Rationale

This initiative enables both the therapist and the client an opportunity to witness how individuals interact with one another. It identifies group dynamics, variations in how individuals relate, and how different dynamics surface in the art process. This experience can be a good first introduction to using nonverbal (art) with clients who may feel resistive or "silly" doing drawings. The free forms and simple lines help to eliminate perceived pressure to produce a "good" drawing.

Personal Comments

Personal comments came from two undergraduate students of Professor Kagin who were not paired but wrote incredible insight into the process.

Figure 5.5 shows a drawing of a bear on the left side with a fish in his paws lifted above his head. A curvilinear line above him creates the suggestion of a mountain range, as further indicated by blue on a mountain top. Dividing the background from the foreground is a purple curvilinear and calligraphic line that suggests the stream from which the fish came. In the foremost, right corner, there is a brown moose standing in green grass. Each section is clearly defined, and sections do not overlap. This image is mentioned in the personal comments of Student One that follow.

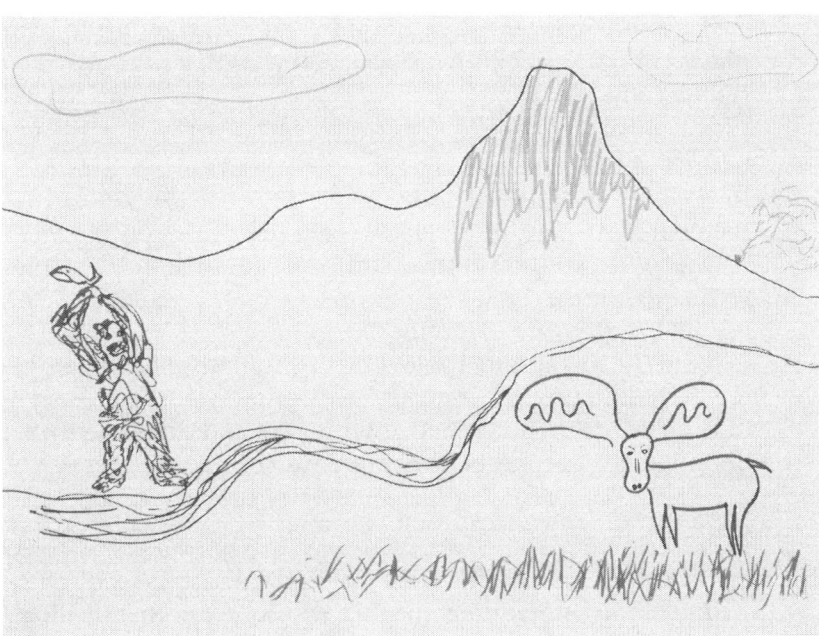

Figure 5.5 Dyadic Nonverbal Communication

Student One

For the first drawing, my partner and I took turns, being careful making intentional marks based on the other person's line. We ended up with a completely representational composition that I drew upside down. I got more and more loose with each partner and I enjoyed it more as I relaxed. I reacted differently to each partner because each pairing had a completely different dynamic.

Therapeutic Transition

This initiative opens up discovery about relationships. This student appears cautious in approaching people she does not know well and takes her cues for her own behavior from them. It would be interesting for the partners to explore the symbolism or significance of the moose, bear, fish, mountain and stream. A good follow-up would be at the Cognitive/Symbolic level, where she was asked to draw a picture of herself in a group and a picture of herself alone. As is indicated in her comments, she was perceptive about the dynamic of each individual and responded accordingly but not in an assertive manner. Having her differentiate her awareness of self within a group and how she perceives herself outside the group would facilitate her understanding of how she engages with others. Explore the difference between the two drawings. Consider elements like size, proximity to others in the group drawing, and difference in configuration of the self. Which was easier to draw, and with which is she more comfortable? Why?

Figure 5.6 shows a series of shapes, some of which have been colored in and some of which are connected to other lines. All of the

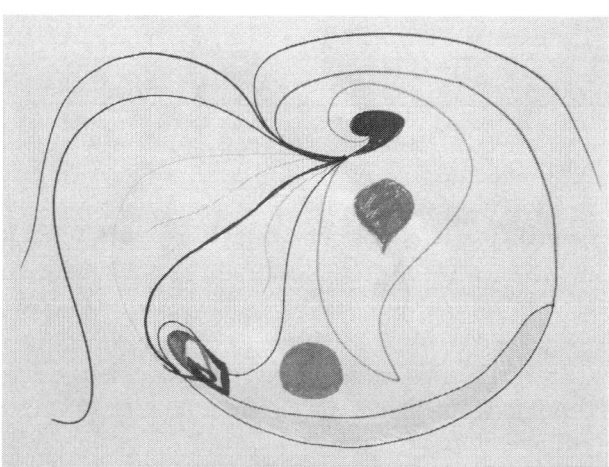

Figure 5.6 Dyadic Nonverbal Communication

shapes and lines seem to radiate from one centralized blue inverted teardrop form near the top third of the drawing.

Student Two
I made it a goal with each partner to make a connection, to make them feel accepted and welcome. I enjoyed moving in unison with my partners. Two of the three really enjoyed and even flourished from the intentionality, while the third partner was freaked out/intimidated by it and retreated. I found it interesting how easy it was to work with some, even easier than individuals I had more of a history with. The way partners felt is evident in the visuals.

Therapeutic Transition

This student, although apparently very much a caregiver, may need to work on her own boundaries and awareness of those of others. Because while she may perceive her actions as intentional and welcoming, the recipient may not always experience them as such. A good initiative for her would be How I See Myself, How Others See Me. Then have the group give her feedback.

Creativity Activation

The creativity level varies in this initiative depending on the interaction of the partners. For some, the creativity level is activated when the person begins to respond and add to the marks of the partner as they think about and make choices that integrate or engage with the partner. For others, creativity level is activated when they problem solve how to communicate nonverbally with the partner. This builds confidence through producing and sharing.

Adaptation

One possible and powerful adaptation for this initiative would be to use clay as the material, which would activate the Kinesthetic/Sensory level, and it would definitely access much more affect. Changing the size of the paper would limit the space for the marks and integration/interaction, causing interpersonal responses to be more contained. The retreating response, as mentioned by Student Two, would be restricted. This would need to be carefully considered by the therapist with respect to the clients and the group dynamics. A change in materials would also elicit different sensory responses, such as pastels that could be blended or moved with hands, and paint, which would be fluid but should only be used with small brushes for control.

Initiative Seven—How I See Myself/How Others See Me

ETC—Perceptual/Affective (P/A) and Cognitive/Symbolic (C/S)
MDV—Low Complexity Unstructured Fluid (LCUF)

Most people have a lot of emotion wrapped up in their perceptions of how others see them and also how they perceive themselves. These can be very sensitive issues, which often present in therapy. This initiative faces this mental construct straight on without much avoidance, as the use of paint allows the affect to flow out onto the page.

Materials

Tempera paint, 2 pieces 18 × 24 drawing paper, various-size brushes, water, paper towels

Directives

1. Using the first sheet of paper, paint how you see yourself.
2. On the second sheet of paper, paint how others see you.
3. Discuss the two paintings. How are they similar? How are they different?

Rationale

This initiative helps the client or student to consider the discrepancies that exist, if any, between their self-perception and how they think others see them. It helps to confront the self and is a good exploration of self-image and self-esteem.

Figure 5.7 shows the image of a female form in brown amid watercolor lines. This is the image for How I See Myself. Figure 5.8 is a watercolor flower-like form of greens, blues, and yellows with a base of reds and browns.

Personal Comments—22-Year-Old Female
Student of Professor Kagin

With how I see myself, I chose a composition I had done before spontaneously that felt very free. When asked to paint how I see myself, this composition came up again. I used yellows and blues to give a motion almost like the wind, driving me forward. These two colors are very spiritual for me, yellow being like Christ's presence and blue being the calm, peacefulness. The figure with her arms above her head is supposed to be me standing almost on a cliff, overlooking something vast and beautiful. The reds and oranges are my

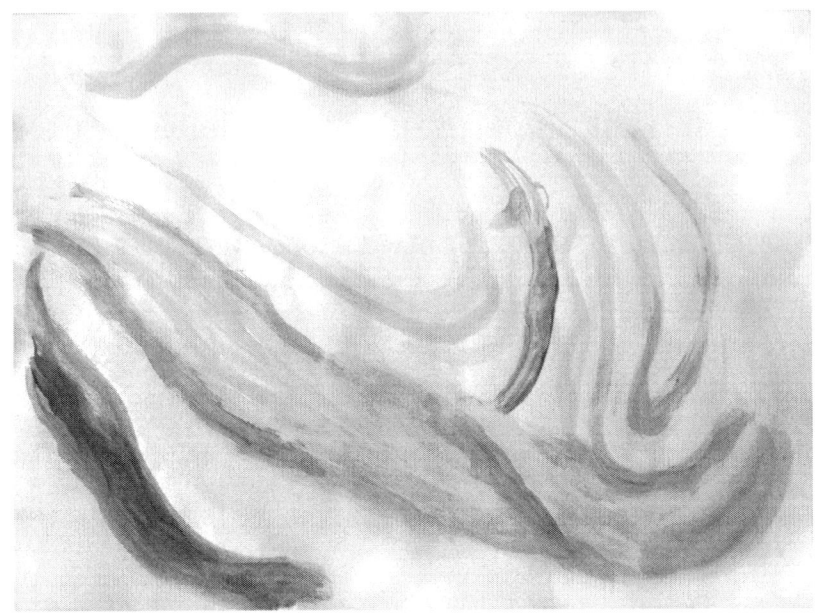

Figure 5.7 How I See Myself

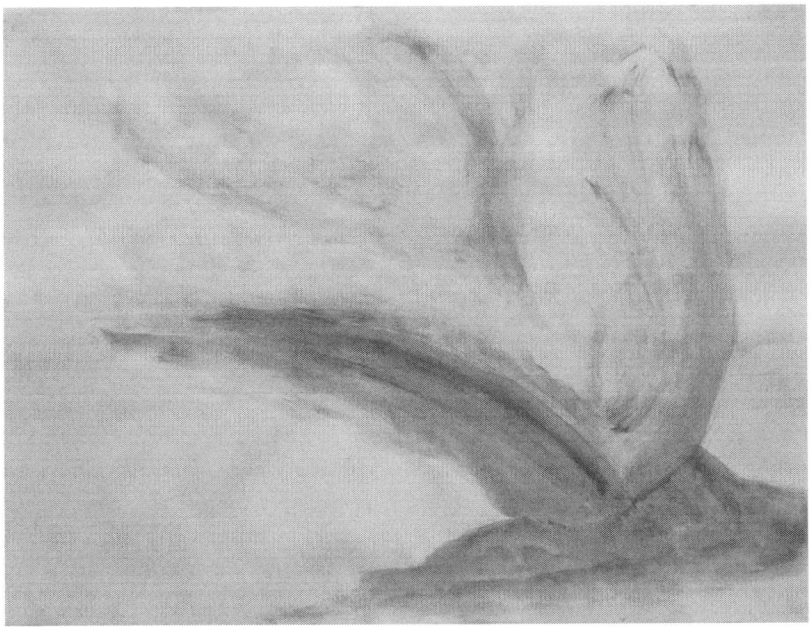

Figure 5.8 How Others See Me

fire, my passions. The browns are representative of being human. I painted myself brown, and included brown throughout the composition. The black and brown in the bottom left are the human but darker parts of myself, the things I do not like about myself but I know are still present. The way I see myself, however these parts do not keep me from being free.

With how others see me, I had more trouble. I thought of something pleasant like a flower, and used my calm blues, lively greens and joyful yellows being what blooms from the flower. That seems to be what most people see. I did not include green in how I see myself, but I did with how others see me. Though the composition of how I see myself is the free and lively one. I put the brown underneath of the flower because it seems like most people don't see the more human side of me, and it gets pushed below the rest. That could be because that's just how people have described me to myself, or because I find it hard to show my more human flawed side with fear that it won't be accepted. But it is the more grounding part of the composition and I see brown as being a very human and grounding color.

Therapeutic Transition

As this student is gaining insight into herself and her behavior toward others, we would encourage further exploration at a more cognitive and concrete level by introducing her to the Box Self, Chapter 6. In contrast to thinking about how others see them, Box Self asks the client to show on the outside of the box what is on the outside of the self. While this is essentially similar information, the cognitive approach changes the response and presents it as what people "see" versus what they "think" even though in this perceptual/affective initiative the term used is *see*. Integrating and processing the two initiatives and their responses would provide great insight.

Creativity Activation

Idea generation is first achieved when participants choose colors for themselves and resonate with the fluidity of materials. This is heightened when clients must think about and paint how others see them, enhancing tolerance for ambiguity as well as sharing with others.

Adaptation

Making changes to the size of the paper can always elicit different responses, so in this case a slightly smaller sheet of paper could contain the affect responses, especially if body image is an issue. Restrictive media could be used for the client who needs more control. This would encourage more of the C/S rather than a full beginning in the P/A. One additional adaptation to this exercise could be the creation of masks for How I See Myself, How Others See Me.

Initiative Eight—Haptic/Visual Self Symbol

ETC—Perceptual/Affective (P/A) and Kinesthetic/Sensory (K/S)
MDV—High Complexity Structured Resistive (HCSR)

The use of clay in this initiative highlights the perceptual affective level of the ETC-MDV, but the process begins at the kinesthetic sensory level. The addition of "I" language and giving voice to the clay form has powerful effects.

Materials

Good-quality (pliable, not too wet and not too dry) clay (white, grey, or red), about a pound or two good handfuls combined; sponges, clay tools, bowl of water, paper towels—if clay tools are not available, use found objects such as a knife, fork, anything textured, screen, toothpicks, or anything at hand. Bowl of water and board or cloth on work table.

Directives

1. Create a self symbol with the clay. Be sure to use both hand work and tools (if desired). Form the symbol with your hands, adding finishing touches with the tools.
2. When completed, look at the piece from all angles and describe what you have done.
3. Then close your eyes and feel the clay, its forms and curves, its ins and outs, its rough edges and smooth. As your hand moves around the clay, describe the exploration with "I am" . ... round, rough, jagged, smooth, etc.
4. Then open your eyes and discuss what has been discovered from the two reflections, haptic and visual.

Rationale

The clay, being three dimensional, assists in creating multiple metaphors and discoveries. Working with the medium alone starts at a kinesthetic/sensory level but soon morphs into form. Pushing, pulling, smoothing, cutting, banging, and all other actions can be absorbed by the media. This absorption often yields emotions as well as a picture of the self at that moment in time. Observing the self creating the self brings questions of who am I today? What do others see that I want to hide or do I actually hide? After the piece is completed, looking at it at every angle and describing what is seen visually promotes memories, emotional reactions, defenses, and intellectualization. Closing the eyes and feeling the piece is an entirely different experience in which you state "I am" and become the piece, in whole and in parts. When that process is complete, there should be new insight and new directions to explore or reinforce whatever needs strengthening, promotes the positive, and leads to the challenges. Stay quietly with the individual as the work is done. Keep the environment as quiet as possible and the lighting appropriate for seeing the work and for introspection.

Figure 5.9 is a natural clay form (freshly formed and pliable). This is the front of the Haptic Visual self created by Author One. Figure 5.10 is the back of the form.

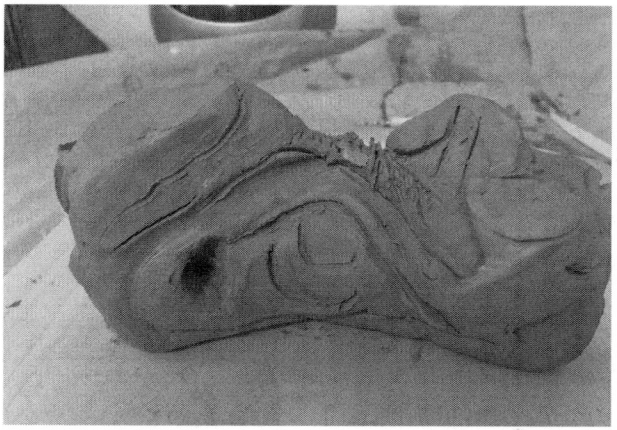

Figure 5.9 Haptic-Visual Self Symbol

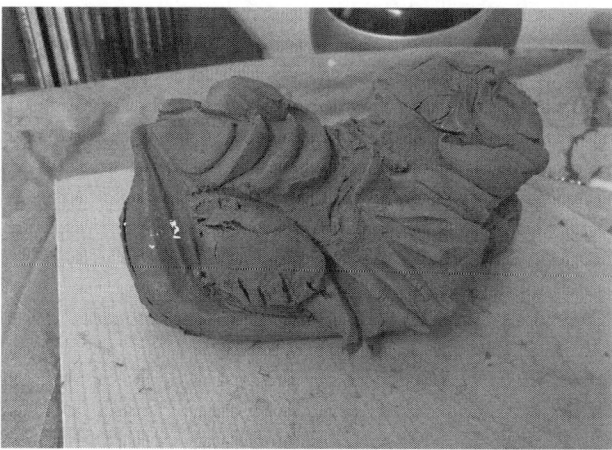

Figure 5.10 Haptic-Visual Self Symbol

Personal Comments—Author One, 72-Year-Old
Professional Art Therapist and Retired Professor

I found my clay to be quite resistive as it was somewhat dried out. But it was pliable enough that I did not need to use too much pressure. I wanted to depict the many aspects and layers of myself in organic form—nothing recognizable but aesthetically pleasing and complex at the same time. I thought of my life now and in the past and attempted to show love and compassion, first for my children, then for others by the inward swirls I created. I also wanted to show the rough edges and depict that I am not "finished" yet. There is still room for growth and renewal. I have been grappling with aging in this decade of my life and find myself thinking a lot of "what ifs"—none of them pleasant. This is the age when friends and family begin to die and we near our life expectancies. My piece has valleys and ridges as if it were created by nature geologically. In many ways this is true. The body changes, the earth sheds and hardens, sagging into crevices that were not there before. But as I turn it there is an intriguing flow, like waves that have washed upon the sand and left their impression. There is a hole, a transparency between the two sides of the piece. I do not know if that is deterioration or insight. Another angle looks like a face or mask with hollow eyes, a big nose and grim features that look scarred. That was my visual description.

Haptic with eyes closed—I am up and down, rough and smooth with no apparent clear direction. I am difficult to navigate as the ridges and texture catch on my fingernails and I must stop to get around them. I have a pathway that begins on the front and stops on the back (order in which I created this) I have a ledge to hold. This side of me is much easier to navigate, I am consistent and directional. When I reach the hole I am delighted to find myself able to get to the other side and am comforted by the round valley I find.

When I opened my eyes and looked at it again it looks very "intestinal" and ancient but full of experience and life. There are places to hide and places to be comforted. When I discover what the rough edges are I know I can smooth them if I desire. I like its differences and its consistencies, its intriguing spaces and its solidness. It is fascinating to me that after I had the haptic experience and combined my perceptions I feel better about the piece, better about me.

Therapeutic Transition

I appear to be in the generative stage of life (Erickson, 1978) in which I am reflecting on my past, integrating my experiences to understand who I am today. At the same time I am facing the reality of mortality.

I was very spontaneous when I began pushing the clay. The forms that resulted from the first kinesthetic reaction were then embellished quite rapidly. I acknowledge impatience and impulsivity and have had to deal with it all my life. Rather than refining the form I continued to create new spaces. I also said I used creative problem solving to fix my mistakes rather than going back and redoing. An initiative that could be suggested to follow up would be to remain at the P/A level and continue clay work but this time be directive, such as make a slab pot and finish it by refining my work. This would help me to see that I am able to slow down and carefully as well as methodically complete a piece.

Figure 5.11 is a plasticine female form in gray with black coils wrapped around it. This was created by a 21-year-old female undergraduate student.

Personal Comments—21-Year-Old Female Undergraduate Student

While creating my self-symbol I didn't really know where I was going with it and how to begin. I started by just manipulating the clay getting used to the texture and trying to get over the weird oily film it left on my hands. Then I began to create a female figure, she was headless and had

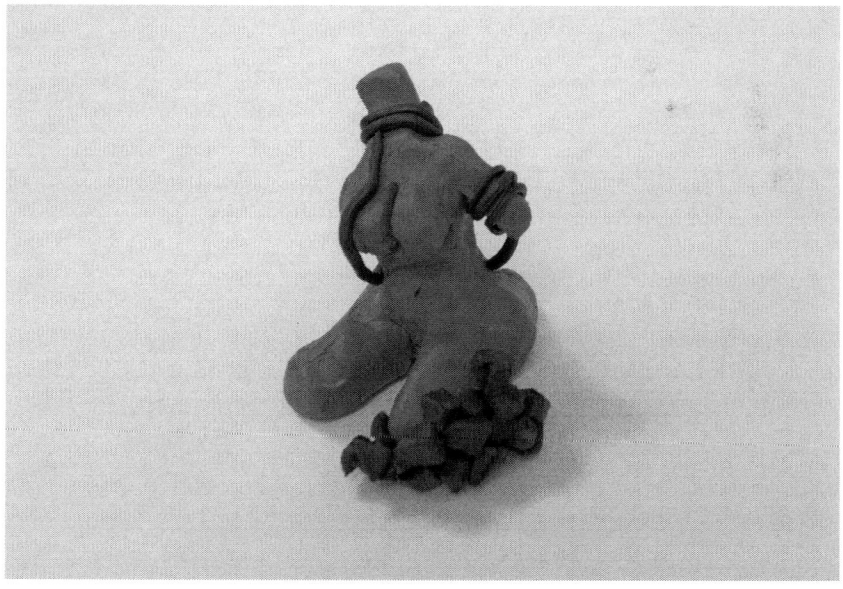

Figure 5.11 Haptic-Visual Self Symbol

over exaggerated hips without feet, calves, or arms. But then something happened inside me. There was a heaviness I could not shake and I began to roll out a coil of black clay and wrapped it around the neck and the arm of the figure, leaving her bound. When asked to describe my symbol to my partner it was uncomfortable for me. Then came time to share with the group and I was anxious because through this process I began to identify what this exercise was showing me about myself. I waited to go last and my comments were short and simple and as I did the Gestalt portion of my description I was fighting back tears. Using the Gestalt language made everything I already knew more real than it has ever been for me. I remember saying the words "I am bound" and that being the moment it really hit me, when it was an object I was safe from it but when it became me it was unavoidable.

Therapeutic Transition

It appears that part of what this young lady is bound by is not fully dealing with her childhood sexual abuse, even though she has been in and out of therapy for many years. Although she has verbally processed her trauma, she has not been fully honest with herself about how this has impacted her life. The manipulation of this form brought out the affective component of her abuse, and the Gestalt (giving voice to it) forced her to say the words she has been unable or unwilling to say.

She is now at a place where she has to decide to choose to remain in bondage or break free. Going to more fluid materials, such as paint, now that she has realized this part of herself will allow her to freely express the emotions of fear, sadness, and anger.

Creativity Activation

Idea generation begins through the sensory experience of forming, touching, and changing the clay. As curiosity builds, so can illumination. There is tremendous intrinsic appeal to this initiative as problem solving and originality coalesce in the producing and then sharing of the experience. Meaning may be further developed when it is integrated symbolically into the haptic and the visual.

Adaptation

In our professional opinion, this initiative is so powerful and sensitive on its own that adaptation is neither necessary nor recommended.

Initiative Nine—Changing Points of View 1

ETC—Perceptual/Affective (P/A) and Cognitive Symbolic (C/S)
MDV—High Complexity Unstructured Fluid (HCUF)

As is common with initiatives on the Perceptual/Affective level of the ETC, the use of paint can be a profound invitation to emotional expression in art. This initiative uses watercolor, which is a very fluid medium. Awareness of the potential increase in vulnerability of the client is important.

Materials

Watercolor paint, various sizes of brushes, three sheets of large watercolor or good drawing paper

Directives

1. Do a painting of how you feel today. This can be about how you feel physically, emotionally, psychologically, or spiritually; or it can represent a life issue.
2. Find a section of the painting that is interesting and create another painting that shows this section enlarged.
3. Create a third painting in which the original painting is reduced or minimized and show the area surrounding the section.
4. Process the transformations.

Rationale

This initiative explores the current affective state or perception of an issue by creating different degrees of reflective distance graphically. Use the paintings as metaphors to discover different aspects of the same emotional/affective state. It allows the client to see varying perspectives (three visuals) and recognize where they are emotionally focused. The use of color in this very fluid experience is also important, and adding color analysis can yield even greater insight.

Figures 5.12 to 5.15 are watercolor paintings by Graves-Alcorn. Figure 5.12 shows blue and violet fluid lines on the bottom and a suggested circular form in yellow at the top. There are four yellow dashes within the blues and violets at the bottom: three on the left and one on the right.

Figure 5.13 is a watercolor close-up of a violet form with fluid and transparent blues and violets surrounding it.

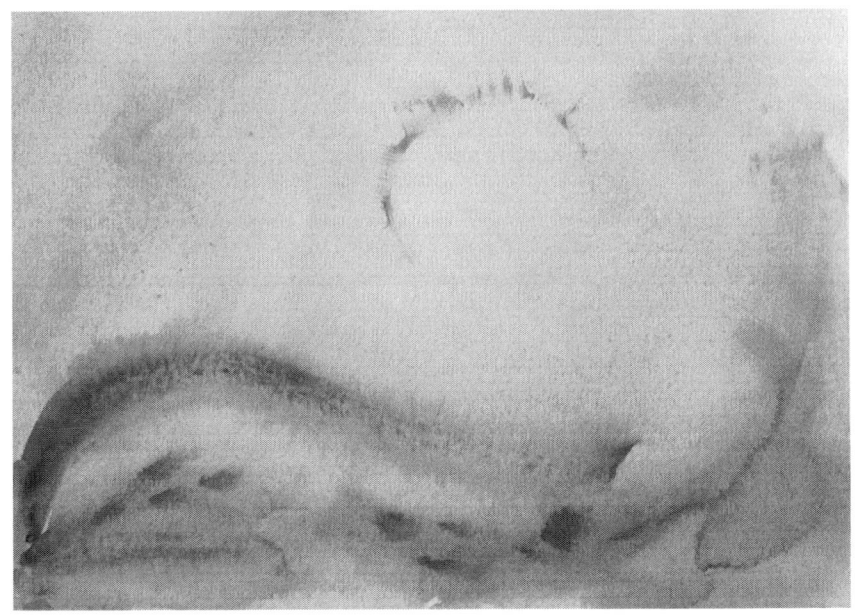

Figure 5.12 Changing Points of View 1 (Painting 1)

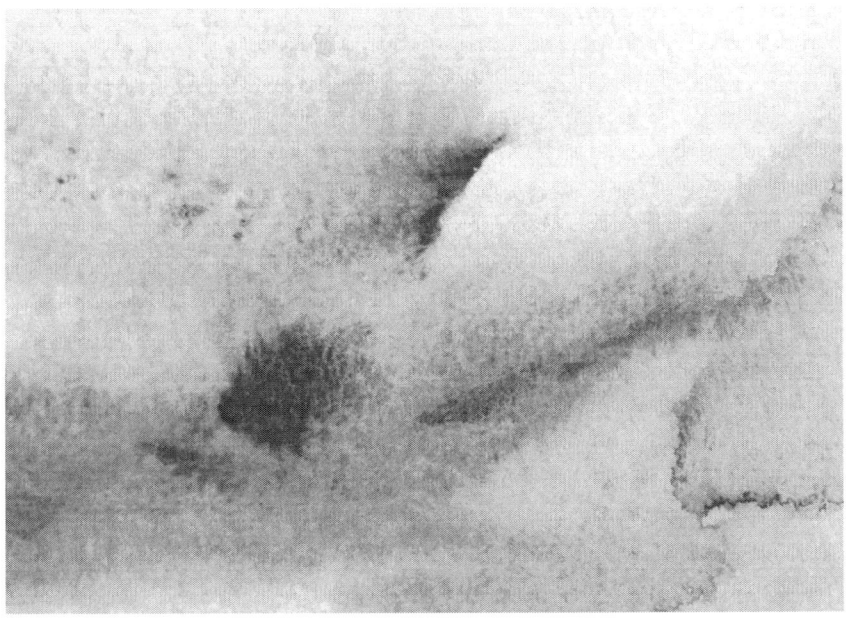

Figure 5.13 Changing Points of View 1 (Close-up)

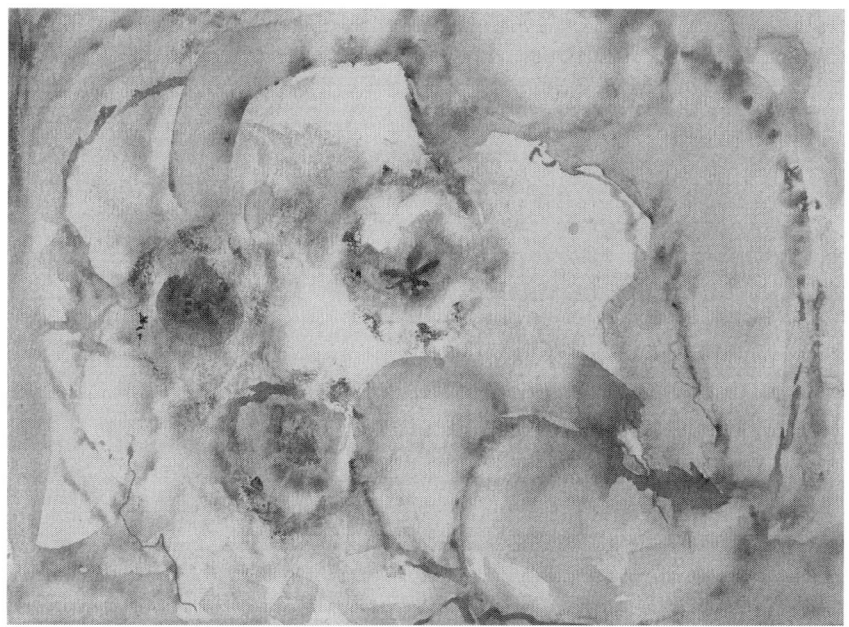

Figure 5.14 Changing Points of View 1 (Painting 2)

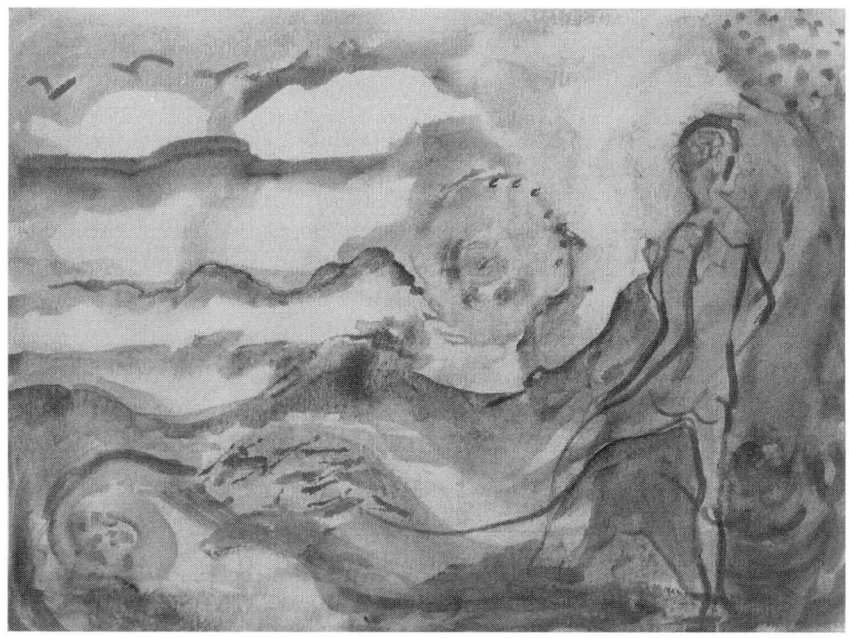

Figure 5.15 Changing Points of View 1 (Painting 3)

Figure 5.14 is a watercolor in blues and violets and some greens. The colors are both saturated and transparent, with a dark-blue star-like form surrounded by violet near the middle.

Figure 5.15 is the final painting by Graves-Alcorn for the Changing Point of View 1 initiative. Represented within it are what appears to be a sun on the horizon over a fluid and watery ground with a female figure in the right corner, looking to the right. Birds and clouds are in the sky on the left of the painting. The same color palette has been used but yellow has been added to this final image.

Personal Comments—Author One, Graves-Alcorn

Painting One
I was feeling very mellow this day, flowing with whatever was happening. I wanted to depict the flow (blue, turquoise and purple) and yellow. I tend to choose these colors often and realize my MARI (Mandala Assessment Research Instrument) training has influenced my expression. Blues tend to represent being in a continual flux, like ocean water. It can also represent intuition and the feminine psyche and role of mother in the world (Takei, 2009). Yellow may indicate the heroic portion of the psyche, and that tends to fit for me. When I put these together they make sense as my life journey has been very full and has had many challenges. I have taken heroic stances and made decisions based upon both mission and intuition. I have also been impulsive and make choices emotionally that were not well thought out. I am who I am today because of both.

Purple relates to past pain and can represent the wounded healer. I believe this is true of most therapists who are willing to examine and introspect. It can be both heroic and painful, but if we continue then so much healing can take place!

Close-Up
I was drawn to this section because it looked like it needed to be "opened" in the blue crevice. Just above the crevice is a dark purple form that is quite prominent.

Painting Two
This painting took me by surprise and as I look at it I see many things, which make some sense to me. The purple has multiplied and scattered, with more intense dark centers of a deep blue. The small star or flower like form radiates in a mandala fashion. If I look at my own process of individuation I realize that the dark blue, which can represent the bad mother, is an area of past memories of my own mother and some guilt over my being a "bad" mother.

It also looks like an arm and fist are either breaking it apart or bouncing it and setting it free. I wonder if the four purple circular shapes represent my four children and the different relationships I have with each. This painting also feels compassionate and caring, like an arm protecting and holding or enfolding. The green areas may represent growth as well. If I look at it from a more Freudian perspective there are prominent phallic symbols as well as those that are more feminine and breast like. I would interpret this in much the same way, a masculine drivenness or power combined with maternal nurturing.

Painting Three—Distancing and Putting in a Greater Context

A figure emerged, looking back and stepping forward. This painting is such an amalgamation of the first two and I really feel it represents me today. I am reviewing my past, but not with resentment and not dwelling on any of the "bruises," but stepping into the flow of feminine intuition and enlightenment. I have been working hard on self-reflection and attempting to change some old patterns. This painting convinces me I really am on my way! It might also represent writing this book! I am pleased that the turquoise (a color associated with healers) is so prominent, as well as the yellow of the horizon into which I am traveling.

Therapeutic Transition—Written by Author Two, Christa Kagin

These images have a congruence from the beginning to the end of the series. The anchor that connects them is the fluidity and the use of line, or lifting out of the line. By the third painting, the lines have come together to produce an image of a power female figure (Author One) who has separated herself and risen above the uncertainties of the watery foundation and horizon. The figure has a solidity, but the ground and the space do not. All of the movement and figural representations face the left (past) and even the body of the woman faces the left; however, her face is turned in a strong but strenuous movement to the right (future). I would encourage her to explore her present by drawing with a resistive medium (graphite or colored pencil) a strong foundation and include her figure somewhere on the foundation. Processing how it feels to see herself on such a stable foundation and what prevents her from actually attaining that would be insightful. She stands strong and heroic, and yet she has portrayed herself in a place that would not support nor allow that in painting three. A comparison of the two paintings would facilitate both an affective and also cognitive symbolic relationship for her to explore.

Creativity Activation

The fluidity of the paint helps resonate fluency and originality. As a close-up is directed, a tolerance for ambiguity must be faced, and then problem solving increases. With each painting, the view is changed and illumination is gained. Personal investment or intrinsic motivation is enhanced.

Adaptations

See Initiative Thirteen—Changing Points of View 2 in Chapter 6, which is adapted from this initiative's directives.

Initiative Ten—Images of Pain and Healing

ETC—Perceptual/Affective (P/A) and Cognitive/Symbolic (C/S)
MDV—High Complexity Unstructured Fluid (HCUF)

This initiative takes two opposite expressions and explores them both individually and together. The integration of contrasting emotions becomes symbolic of acceptance and resiliency.

Materials

Offer a choice of paint (watercolor, tempera, or acrylic) and several size brushes or oil pastels, three pieces of drawing or watercolor paper of equal size

Directives

1. Relax into a comfortable position and become aware of your breathing, paying attention to taking breath in and letting it out.
2. Imagine a flow of soft light traveling inside your body, from your head to your toes. Slowly be aware of each area examined.
3. Allow whatever thoughts and feelings you may have to simply exist.
4. Imagine your pain, your sense of being overwhelmed as a color and a form.
5. Select your colors and brush size and paint or draw your image.
6. Set this painting or drawing aside.
7. Imagine the colors and form of healing energy.
8. Paint or draw those colors and forms on a second piece of paper.
9. Put it aside.
10. Contemplate the two images. Do not judge, just observe. Be with them in a mindful manner, exploring all nuances you have created.
11. Close your eyes and breathe into your body, recognizing any tension, pain, fear, sadness you may experience. Let it go.
12. Pick up a third piece of paper and paint your healing surrounding or breaking apart or integrating with your pain. Paint this image.
13. Lay the three images side by side. What do you observe?

Rationale

We all need a perspective on our experiences. This initiative provides the opportunity to focus on the pain and healing separately but mandates the integration of the two. Work with processing each image. Ask how the colors reflect the experience, or do they? If not, explore why. How powerful and soothing is the image of healing? Process those forms and colors and compare them with those depicted of pain.

Note the size and use of space. Does this reflect an overall pattern of coping with painful feelings?

Concentrate on the third integrative painting. If the individual is satisfied with the painting, let it be. If not, ask "what if?" questions about size, shape, color, amount of space used. What if this part or that part of the healing were larger, smaller, lighter, darker? Your clinical judgment is crucial here, as you wish to guide, not project.

This particular initiative is very helpful following a major loss or trauma, when the individual feels overwhelmed and has trouble identifying the emotions. It may be important to review the function of anger, sadness, fear, and happiness as our bodies seek homeostasis, adaptation, and resilience. It is also important to remember that physical and emotional pain are often interchangeable.

Figure 5.16 shows a star-like form in gold and silver that is the Image of Pain, created by Graves-Alcorn. In the center there is a black oval from which all other marks radiate. The silver is contained within the gold marks and shapes.

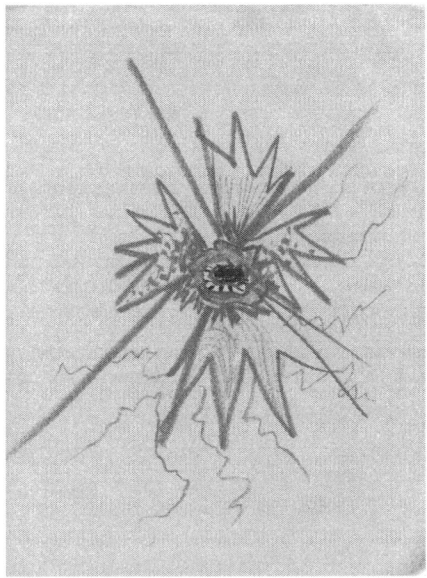

Figure 5.16 Images of Pain and Healing (Image of Pain)

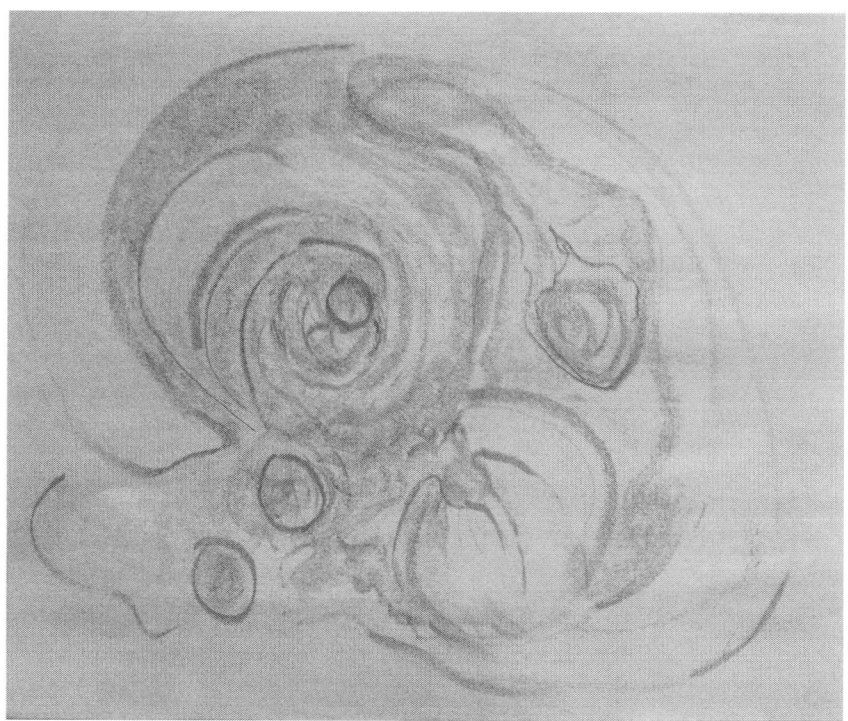

Figure 5.17 Images of Pain and Healing (Image of Healing)

Figure 5.17 is the Image of Healing from Initiative Ten. It is a fluid form that resembles a brain, with five distinct circles within green, violet, blue, and pink lines and colors.

Figure 5.18 is the Image of Healing Integrated with Pain. This shows a flower or amoeba-like form in pink with greens and blues in the center. All of the form is filled with color.

Personal Comments—Author One, Graves-Alcorn
Drawing One—When I drew this I was in physical pain. My left hip and right knee were calling attention to my body. We had also been writing this book and sitting for hours without a break, which is not too smart, so I think I had some anger going on also. Noting the sharp points radiating from a dark "kernel" in the center, there are also lines that look like they are emanating energy. It looks the way I was feeling both physically and emotionally.

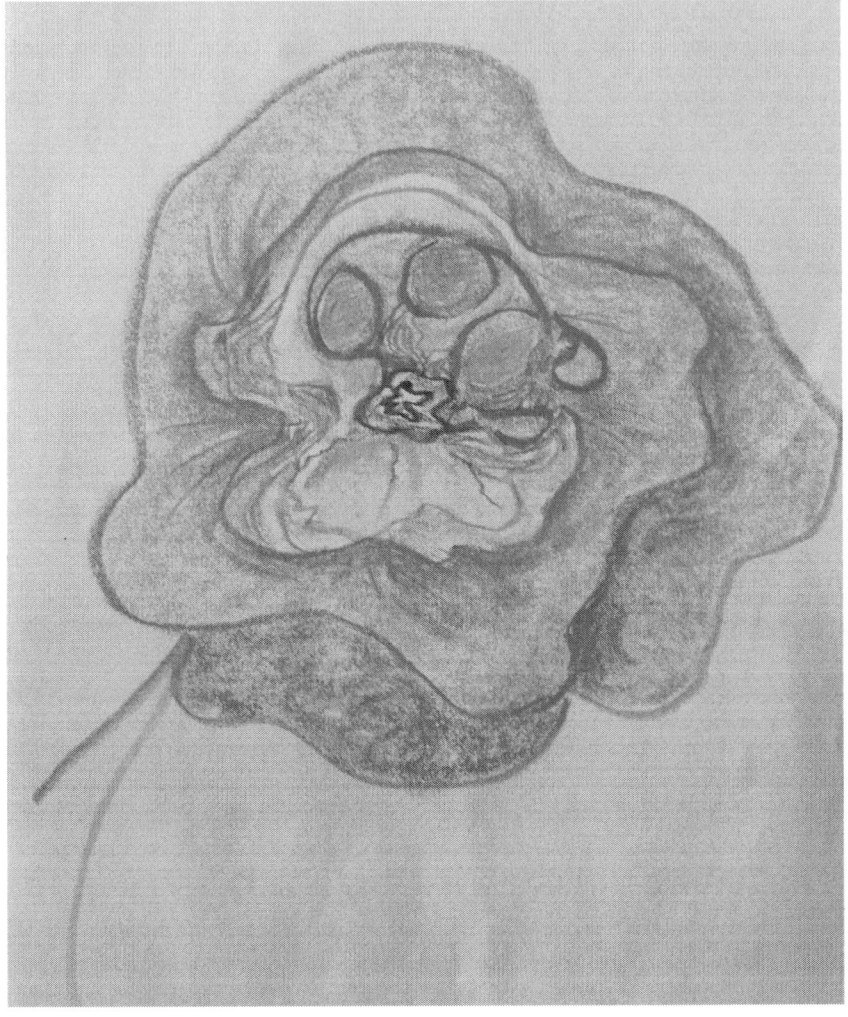

Figure 5.18 Images of Pain and Healing (Image of Healing Integrating with Pain)

Drawing Two—All I could think of was curling up into something soft and being held and soothed. The colors and curvilinear forms remind me of compassion and nurturing.

Drawing Three—This surprised me as I was once again in pain from sitting and writing all day, but had some wonderful experiences with my coauthor which were also very enlightening. She was nurturing me! The image became a flower, the kernel of pain being the seed into which the plant blooms. I realized that there are times when I am so independently stubborn that I do not allow the soothing of others, or myself. This was a very therapeutic experience.

Therapeutic Transition, by Graves-Alcorn

Since I discovered this about myself, the next step for me would be to become more mindful of my own body and how I ignore it at times and taking better care of myself. The other therapeutic intervention would be to insist on asserting myself and ask others for help or a hug. My coauthor also noted the "zygote"-like symbols which were both male and female. Perhaps the birthing of this book and acceptance of this generative stage of my life are incubating. She also noted the whole image looks like a brain with a stem. That is interesting to me, as my childbearing years are behind me and I am renewing my academic and scholarly life. Therapeutically, it is important for me to continue my art, keep my mind active, and exercise.

Creativity Activation

Creativity in this initiative focuses on idea generation as the fluidity of the medium resonates and activates an illuminated state of insight. The ambiguity of word and form that need problem solving integration often yields originality and diversity in thinking. Resiliency occurs with the realization that pain is the path to enlightenment and healing.

Adaptation

This initiative could easily be adapted by changing the media used, such as mixed media and even clay. Additionally, the pain drawing could be completed on paper, while the healing could be completed on a transparency sheet. When finished, the transparency could be placed over the top of the pain so the client could actually see the healing over it. Then the client could have the option of creating a final integrated drawing or processing from this point.

Initiative Eleven—Mandala, the Great Round

ETC—Perceptual/Affective (P/A) and Cognitive/Symbolic (C/S)
MDV—Low Complexity Unstructured Resistive (LCUR)

The circle has been universally accepted as a religious image of perfection, a shape of total symmetry, hermetically closed off from its surroundings. It is the most general shape, possessing the fewest individual features but serving at the same time as the matrix of all possible shapes.

—Rudolph Arnheim, *Visual Thinking* (1983, p. 17)

We highly recommend you read Carl Jung's book *Mandala Symbolism* (1973). It is also recommended that the reader takes the courses (seminars) on the MARI or other expert training in the mandala.

Suzanne Fincher, author of several workbooks on the mandala (2009) states, "mandalas offer us a profound way to examine our inner reality, to integrate that understanding with our physical selves, and to feel connected to the greater universe" (2009, p. 1). In other words, the mandala is a holistic body–mind–spirit initiative. Also, "coloring" the mandala has a positive effect on negative stress.

When coloring, we activate different areas of our two cerebral hemispheres, says psychologist Gloria Martínez Ayala in an interview with Elena Santos of *The Huffington Post* (2014). She states, "The action involves both logic, by which we color forms, and creativity, when mixing and matching colors. This incorporates the areas of the cerebral cortex involved in vision and fine motor skills [coordination necessary to make small, precise movements]." She goes on to explain that activity is lowered in the amygdala as a result of the relaxation brought on by coloring which thereby can impact the way stress is experienced (Santos, 2014). Since our emotions are controlled by the amygdala, the decreased activity can provide for a sense of relaxation. Mandalas have become popular in recent American culture in the form of coloring books with intricate designs and have flooded the market. While we know these to be helpful and meditative for some, we feel the act of working to create within your own circle, untouched by another's ideas, to be of the most benefit to the client and student.

Materials

A circular template such as a 9-inch pie plate, square scrapbooking paper, oil pastels

Directives

1. Here is a circle.
2. This circle is a universal symbol for life and the self.
3. Using the oil pastels (demonstrate if necessary to show the ability to blend), create your mandala by using line, form, and color.

Rationale

Because this initiative is so informative, it is often one of the first things done after an intake. In fact, it is an excellent assessment instrument if you are trained in the MARI. If not, it gives a reference point throughout therapy and is a very revealing/healing instrument in itself. The client is always asked to comment and look at each mandala as a metaphor of his/her world at that moment. It is also useful for children and teens.

Figure 5.19 shows a mandala with vibrant greens, purples, blues, reds, and yellows surrounding multiple eyes. There is an oval near the top left and a green ellipse just below it marking what appears to be a horizon.

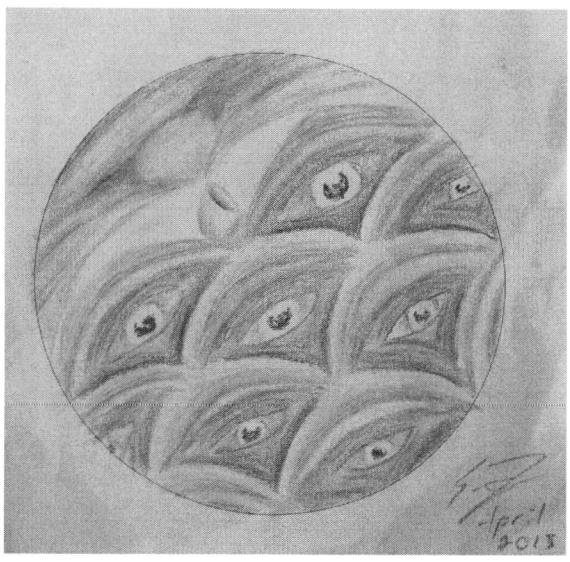

Figure 5.19 Mandala, the Great Round

Personal Comments—43-Year-Old Male

This man was in recovery for addiction to alcohol and drugs and had just returned from a month of spiritual seeking with a shaman in Peru. The colors and symbols contained herein are potent and rich.

The most prominent and frequently used symbol in this mandala is the eye. Referring to *The Book of Symbols: Reflections on Archetypal Images* (Ronnberg and Martin, 2010), the eye is multivalent and can represent God, insight, paranoia, wisdom. It can also represent the totality of consciousness.

When this man was working with the Shaman and using native herbal medicine, he experienced an incredible vision of the universe and its connections to everything (matter and energy). He saw a "creature" from another dimension that was a large eye. They gazed at each other with full acceptance before the eye flew away. It is fascinating that the "single eye" symbol can represent a unity of vision (Ronnberg and Martin, 2010, 354) in which the inner and outer self are resolved.

"Seen more obliquely, the eye corresponds metaphorically to initiation, to fleeting visions of beauty, the spirits of things, the emotional center of a storm, the essentials of experience and the secrets of the soul" (Ronnberg and Martin, 2010, 354). The shadow side of these secrets can result in paranoia and deep fears.

The colors this man chose are also highly significant. First, they are consistently clear and bright, associated with the limbic system (feelings), and indicate a relationship with the world in which creativity overcomes struggle. The yellows indicate the hero's journey, while the reds indicate passion and high energy. Blue is an intuitive color and often associated with spirituality and the feminine. The greens may represent the healing that has taken place, and the purple can be the color of the wounded healer and also relates to a feeling of specialness. The arches seen throughout are also associated with transcendence and entering another stage of growth, consistent with the somewhat "fetal" shapes inside the eyes, which are associated with beginnings. At the time he did this drawing, he was very much at peace with himself.

Therapeutic Transition

The most salient feature of this mandala is the numerous eyes. Since these are multivalent symbols and can represent the dichotomy or paradox of wisdom and paranoia, we would recommend focusing on drawing what one eye "sees." Another initiative would be Changing Points of View, in which the interior of the eye (the iris and pupil) was explored close up and then put into a "far away" context. Continuation of drawing mandalas is also highly recommended.

Creativity Activation

The creativity activation begins with the first mark on the blank circle and continues throughout the process. Each individual will begin differently; some will draw the circle and begin to fill it, while some will draw the circle and pick up a new tool to begin to fill the circle, and still others will begin by writing. Regardless of this first mark and action sequence, creativity is activated when the challenge of "what to put inside" is presented. Each decision will initiate another action, resulting in a creative flow.

Figure 5.20 is a mostly blue circle with a yellow center.

Personal Comments—Author Two, Christa Kagin
I did not learn about the mandala as much through graduate school as I did during my travels and my own research. I studied Hindu shrines, Buddhist stupas, the history of the Labyrinth, and art historical references as the art and architecture of world cultures tells us much about the people of those

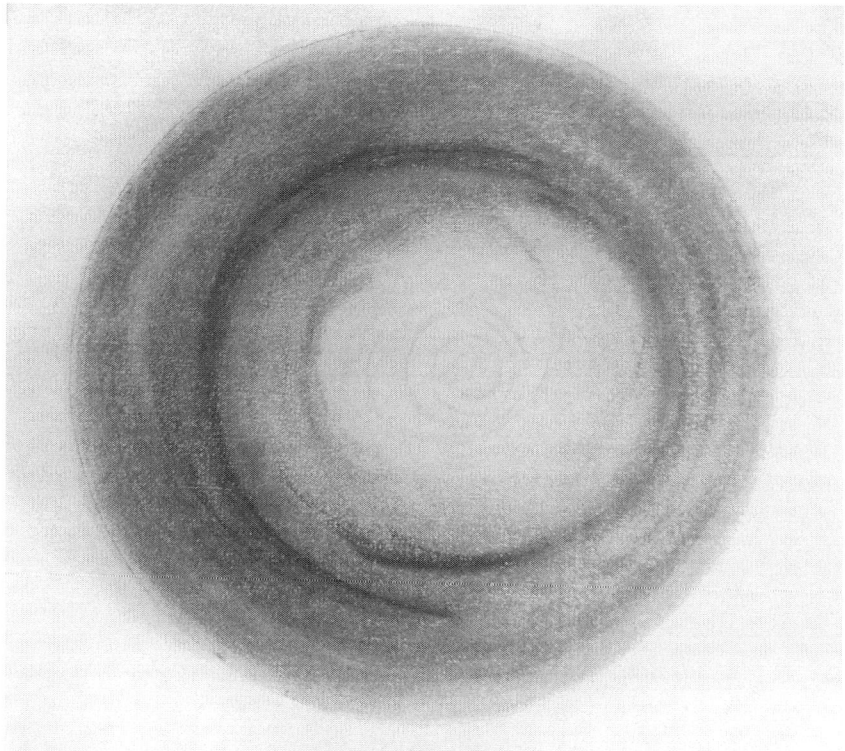

Figure 5.20 Mandala, the Great Round

cultures. Much has been carried down through the ages and is as pertinent today as it was in ancient times. Symbology of the circle is significant globally. Whether it is a physical act of walking in a meditative circle, focusing your eyes within a circle in prayer, participating in rituals in a physical circle of people or drawing a circle yourself, humanity has long understood the centering and healing power of the round.

In my classroom as well as therapy sessions, I use the mandala as a homework assignment. Also I have the person draw their own circle rather than use a template. I ask the person to reflect upon the size of the circle, its placement on the page, whether or not they remained within the boundary and was the whole space filled or is there both positive and negative use of space, giving consideration to the colors and lines used. Discussion of the formal elements and how these become metaphors for the self evolves naturally. The processing can be completely different if you have not had the MARI training. It is stressed rather that mandalas are a meditative experience and have been used for centuries by indigenous peoples. The circle is representative of wholeness and is spiritual in nature. I encourage several mandalas over time.

When students are struggling with creativity and feeling blocked, I ask them to create a mandala focusing on the fact that there are no rules or requirements, only that something goes in. Sometimes when they are stressed I ask them to draw the circle, fill the exterior space with burdens, stress, etc. and then to breathe and fill the inner circle with all the positivity they have. This creates a visual of protection for that which is good and untouched by the stress. If they are struggling with something personal I have them write a word lightly in the middle of the mandala and then work over the top of the word so it is gone and replaced with something that is centering.

I teach undergraduate fine art and art history as well as art therapy, and ask all my students in every class to do at least one mandala. It has become something of a badge of honor to the student who receives the instruction, showing the potency and potential of the circle. The literature reveals that mandalas are calming and focusing for children in classrooms as well. The act of doodling or drawing helps to facilitate retention of knowledge, development of creativity and positive awareness of self. There are numerous mandala coloring books or templates for both children and adults on the market today.

Therapeutic Transition—by Author One, Graves-Alcorn

There are two aspects of this mandala that stand out and are very informative: the color and the concentricity of form. At the stage of beginning to acquire knowledge, epistemology, psychic energy, and heightened consciousness, this symbol especially attends to the urge to awaken and desire for a path and direction. How appropriate for a woman of Christa's stature and age!

I was especially taken with her color choice. Several shades of blue and turquoise are prominent, indicating an ability to relate to others in a mature way and an openness to others' differences. It also indicates growing autonomy, receptivity, and intuition. The light blue that surrounds the mandala may indicate a sense of trust that has developed out of trouble or trauma. It is also indicative of healing. The medium blue heightens intuitive understanding of the self, and the dark blue indicates there are challenges remaining that involve the depths of the unconscious, the "bad" mother (or critical parent), being judged, and the heaviness of that experience. Countering those feelings, however, is the core of yellow and gold, the color of the birth of the hero and fulfillment of a mission (Takei, 2009). The purples are the colors of bruises, of which the healing nature of the color turquoise attests. Therapists and caregivers tend to choose the turquoise shades. She was pleased with her mandala.

I would ask her to confront her challenges directly and suggest using the Battle Drawing as the next initiative (Chapter 6).

Creativity Activation

When the client begins the process of moving hand and media into the circle, developing a figure–ground relationship, creativity is activated. From this point, the definition of the whole elicits a full immersion in the process. The circle is a challenge but also a container, a natural place for creativity to flourish and for the client to center and focus, leaving weight of struggle or finding clarity of mind.

Adaptation

The following adaptations are used by Professor Kagin in several of her classes:

There are many adaptations to this directive. I have employed all of the adaptations listed in this section, either with clients or with students in the art therapy specialization courses or in studio courses. Of all of the "extra" activities I have assigned, these centered around variations on the mandala have proven to be the most impactful to students, and sometimes, long after they have graduated, they send me notes to tell me about mandalas they have drawn or send links to images. This is a testimony to the power they have in multiple applications.

Figures 5.21, 5.22, and 5.23 are pastel-drawn mandalas on black paper. Figures 5.24, 5.25, and 5.26 are mandalas drawn on white paper. In each of these mandalas, the circle was drawn as part of the initiative rather than using a template. Furthermore, each is different, highlighting the diversity and inventiveness brought forth by this seemingly simple action.

Visual Word Mandala—Used Primarily in Studio Courses

Depending on the challenge being faced, determine whether you need to open up your mind and thoughts to flow freely or if you need to center and push out distractions to come to a clarity of mind. If it is opening up, you will begin in the middle and work your way out in a circular pattern. If it is focusing you need, you will begin on the outside of the page and work your way to the middle in a circular pattern. Begin with a word, the first word that comes to mind or a word associated with the challenge or need. Begin then to alternate between word and image or mark. Word. Image. Word. Image. Use free association when working. Don't force a word or image but rather let your mind be free to go where it will. (Sometimes these have more images than words and vice versa.)

I have found that these mandalas often provide just the insight needed or exactly the freedom sought to move students to the next step in a project, the formulation of a concept for painting or drawing, to address a creative block or guide them in a personal challenge. They even assign them to each other now!

Dual Mandalas with Contrast

Another variation of the mandala that has been used with students and also clients is the production of two mandalas in a single sitting utilizing soft pastels and another medium of choice on black and white paper, respectively. The soft pastels on black paper are a favorite because the color pops off of the page and the black creates a strong contrast with the color marks made. Furthermore, the softness of blending or moving the soft pastels across the black paper creates a dimension in the circle.

Following are examples of mandalas produced by students. The mandalas on white paper (Figures 5.24, 5.25, and 5.26) were created with marker or oil pastel, a choice offered to them. The ones on black paper (Figures 5.21, 5.22, and 5.23) are created with soft pastels. As previously mentioned, the movement of the pastel across the black page produces a dimension in the circle. Contrasting the white mandalas, you can see that the marks appear simply as marks on the page and a circle with marks or colors within it. However, the black paper

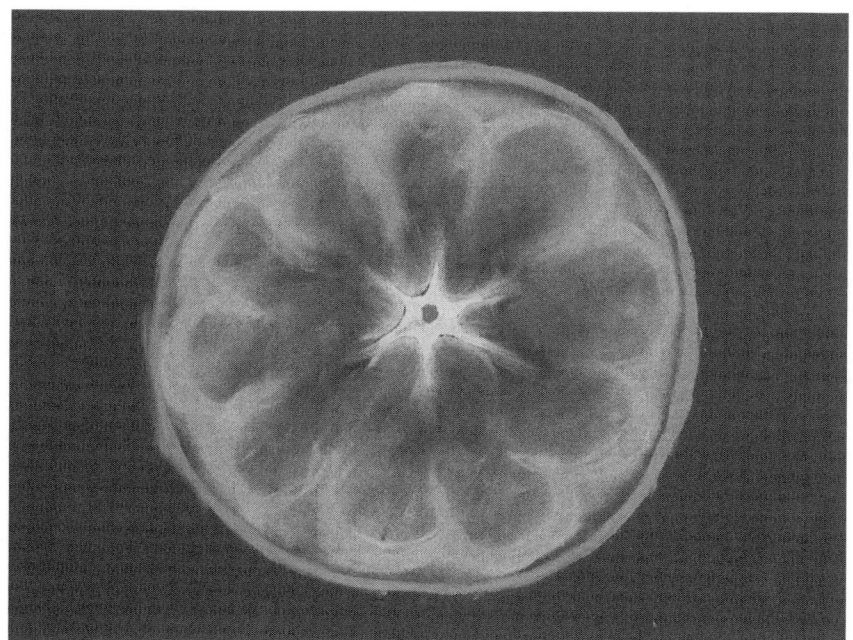

Figure 5.21 Mandala, the Great Round

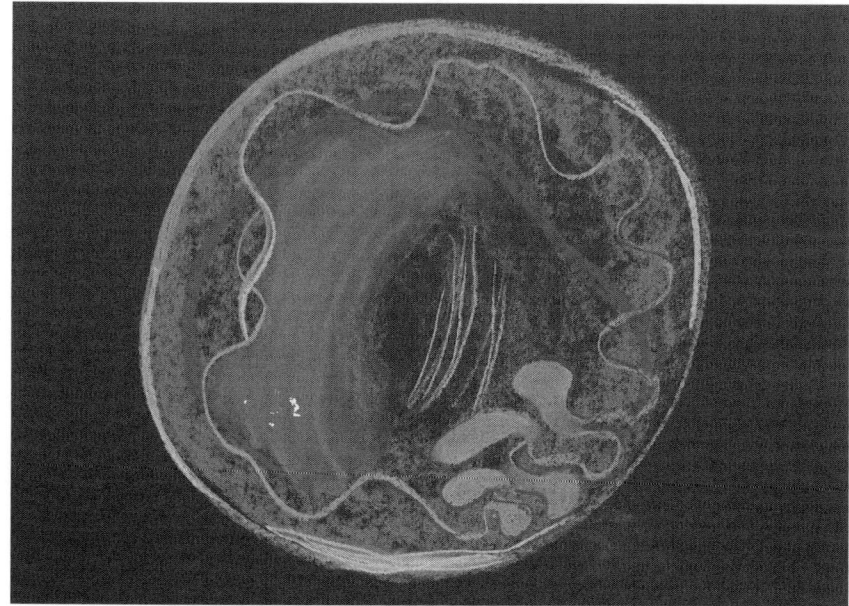

Figure 5.22 Mandala, the Great Round

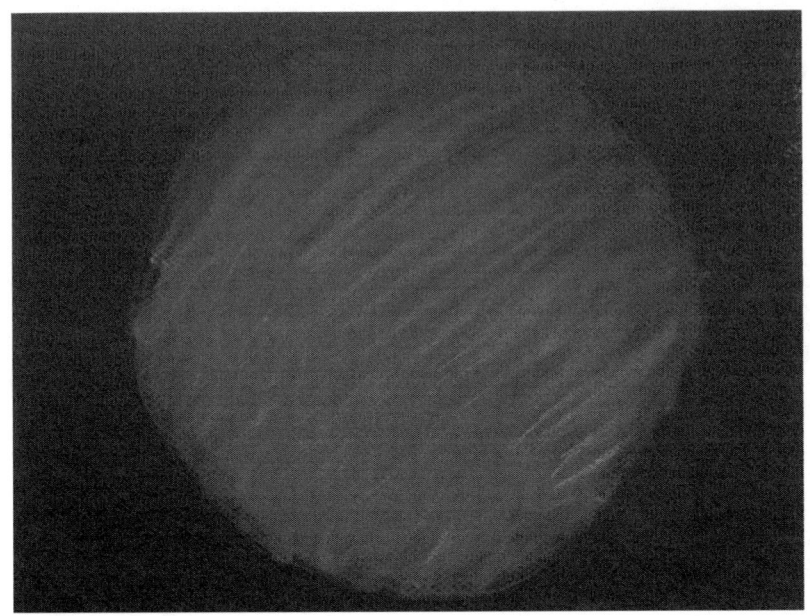

Figure 5.23 Mandala, the Great Round

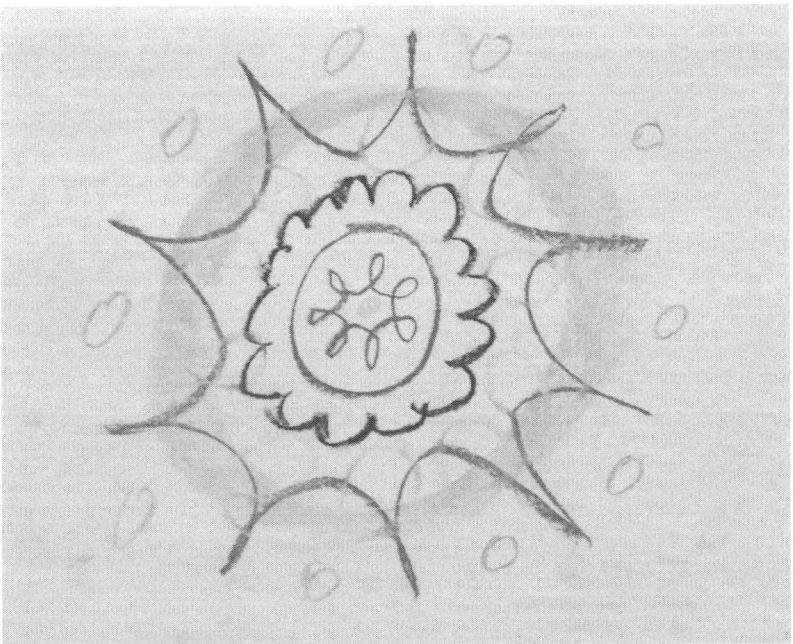

Figure 5.24 Mandala, the Great Round

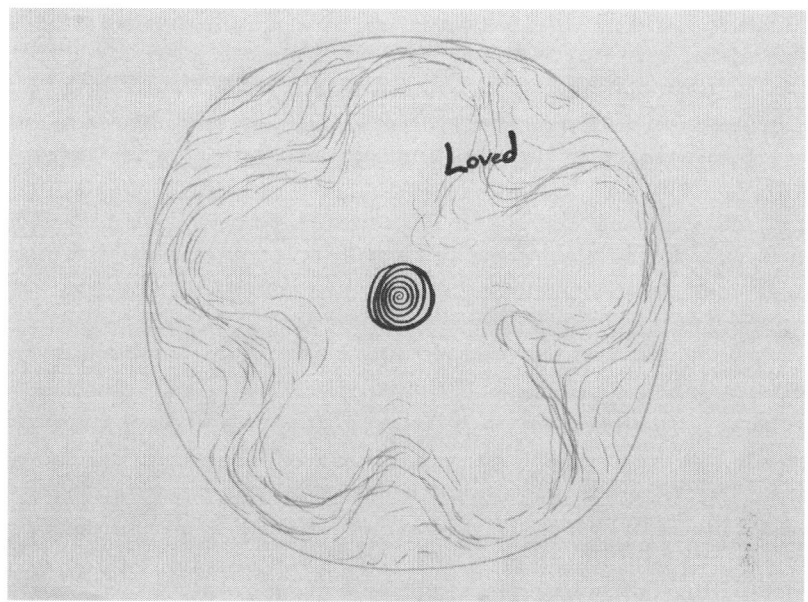

Figure 5.25 Mandala, the Great Round

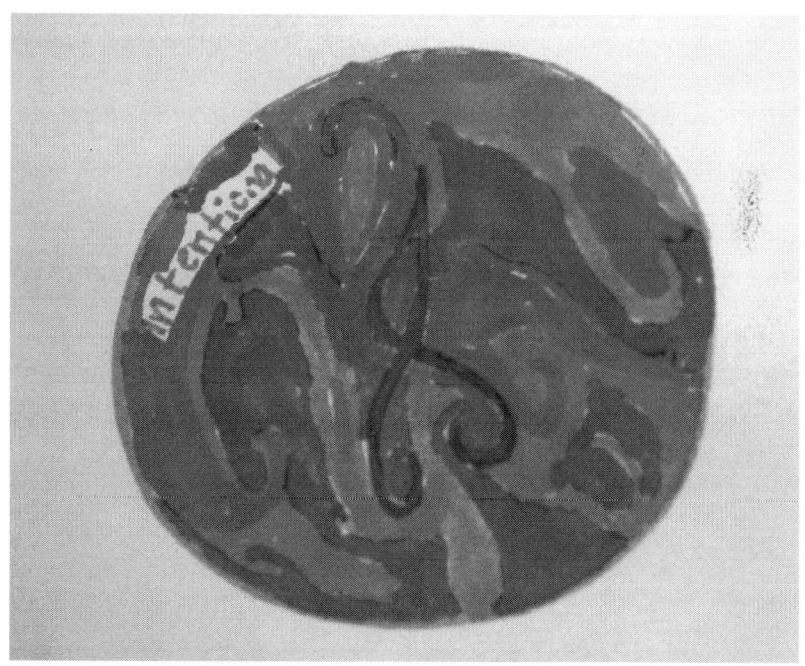

Figure 5.26 Mandala, the Great Round

contrasts so strongly with the pastel that the smudging with fingers creates a haze. This can produce an imprecise image, a glowing effect, and even the suggestion of movement (see Figure 5.23). While still simply marks on the paper, the contrast of the black with the color and the ways it can be seen "through" the color suggest a space, a void, an opening, a form "on" the page or receding inward. This small adaptation creates a provocative image that creators respond to and reflect on deeply. The boldness of the color and the distinctions within the textures of the marks create an encounter for the client that is unlike the mandala on the white page.

Word-Insertion Mandala

Additionally, the insertion of the word in a circle and then marks to complete the mandala can create a centering that is directed rather than left to the client or student to solve unto themselves. In the mandala image in Figure 5.25, the word "loved" is written in purple. This was created following the directive to draw a circle (freehand), write a positive affirmation *word* in the mandala, and then complete it. The lines move over the word but do not cover it. The form within the circle is flowerlike and includes a spiral in the center. The lines radiating off of the flower to the edge of the circle suggest movement and ripples like water. It was a positive image that was centering and affirming.

Figure 5.24 was created with the directive to draw a mandala. Left to create the whole circle and image in a completely unstructured way, this mandala makes use of the page fully, and although the points of the form move outside of the primary gray circle, they are surrounded by smaller circles (ovals) that create a radiating pattern. This repetitious mandala has been created in layers with multiple circular marks, and though they are not all simply circles, they do maintain the integrity of the mandala's centering power to create cohesion. Not only does the circle contain something within it (flowerlike forms layered together), it also appears to produce a spontaneous and yet orderly release. All of these elements create opportunities for the client to explore the give and take in life and the passive and active roles currently being experienced.

References

Agell, G. (1998). Rita Simon: An interview with a founder of art therapy. Editor. *American Journal of Art Therapy*, 36 (3), 68. American Art Therapy Association.

Arnheim, R. (1983). *The Power of the Center: A Study of Composition in the Visual Arts*. Berkeley & Los Angeles, CA: University of California Press.

Dondis, D. (1973). *A Primer of Visual Literacy*. Cambridge, MA & London, UK: The Massachusetts Institute of Technology Press.

Erickson, E. (Ed.) (1978). *Adulthood: Essays*. New York, NY: Norton & Company.

Fincher, S. (2009). *The Mandala Workbook: A Creative Guide for Self-Exploration, Balance and Well-Being*. Boston & London: Shambhala.

Jung, C. (1973). *Mandala Symbolism*. Princeton, NJ: Princeton University Press.

Rhyne, J. (1974). *The Gestalt Art Experience*. Chicago, IL: Magnolia Street Publishers.

Rhyne, J. (1979). *Drawings as Personal Constructs: A Study in Visual Dynamics*. Unpublished doctoral dissertation, UMI dissertation services, Ann Arbor, Michigan.

Ronnberg, A. (Ed. in chief) and Martin, K. (Ed.) (2010). *The Book of Symbols: Reflections on Archetypal Images*. Cologne, Germany: Taschen.

Santos, E. (2014). Coloring Isn't Just for Kids. *The Huffington Post*. Retrieved from http://www.huffingtonpost.com/2014/10/13/coloring-for-stress_n_5975832.html.

Scheerer, M. and Lyons, J. (1957). Line drawings and matching responses to words. *Journal of Personality*, 25, 251–273.

Takei, M. (2009). MARI: The Great Round. Raleigh, NC: Mandala Assessment Research Institute.

CHAPTER 6

Cognitive-/Symbolic-Focused Initiatives

This chapter presents initiatives that emphasize the cognitive and symbolic functions of the expressive therapies continuum. You will note that the majority of the initiatives are included in this chapter because they are generally the most often used in the therapeutic setting and are more complex, as they make use of the K/S and P/A as components.

We now turn to the cortex as our focus. Ultimately behavior change rests on awareness, knowledge, insight, and problem solving, yielding some action at all five levels of being human, the physical, emotional, intellectual, spiritual, and social. A change of patterns is appropriate throughout life. Resilience depends on the ability to adapt, accept, grieve change and move forward with fresh motivation. Biologically, our cells are altered minute by minute. We need to figure out how to keep up with ourselves!

Initiative Twelve—The Word

ETC LEVEL—Cognitive/Symbolic (C/S)
MDV—High Complexity Structured Resistive (HCSR)

We encounter and use words every day. Often we don't realize the power given or not given to the words we use. This initiative explores the use of words, the meaning we impose, and the meaning we extract but applies this awareness in an abstract way to foster this awareness.

Materials

Markers, 8 ½ × 11 paper, glue stick or rubber cement, words cut out of magazines, pastels or markers

Directives

Before the group meeting, have someone objectively cut words from a variety of magazines. Choose various sizes, colors, fonts, and words. This should not be the therapist or the teacher who chooses the words. Put them in an envelope.

Pass around the envelope of words cut from magazines. Without looking, each group member will choose four words.

1. Each person will read the words and think about them. Each person will choose the word that will be a goal.
2. Glue the first word to the page anywhere.
3. Once each person has finished, they will choose a word that is opposite or distant from the first word; perhaps it doesn't relate.
4. Glue the second word onto the page, thinking about the distance.
5. Next, each group member must trade one of the two remaining words with someone in the group.
6. Now add one of the words between the two words already present on the collage. It can be a barrier between the words.
7. Finally, add the fourth and final word to the page.
8. Complete the collage by adding and/or changing with the pastels and markers.
9. Process the words: how they were chosen to be used, what meaning was assigned to them, how they can relate and not relate. How does this exercise make you become aware? How does it interrupt your way of seeing what you thought you were doing?

Rationale

Because the words are not chosen by the client but rather randomly received as he or she reaches into an envelope and pulls out four words, the client must begin to work with what is given. Each person will assign meaning to the words as they move forward with the exercise. As this happens, beliefs, emotions, thoughts of self, and resistance will all be present. With each additional step given after completing the previous one, choices must be made to move forward with the words that have been received. This exercise forces the client to deal with what he/she has in an abstract, external way while deciding how to use the given words. Creating a division or barrier and then completing the entire collage with added materials facilitates problem solving. It becomes apparent as the person works to complete the collage. His or her choice of meaning applied to the words is very personal and enhances free association. What seemed to be unrelated and distant in the beginning has now become a personal statement.

Figure 6.1 is a collage made up of words and color. The two most visible words are Inspired (middle of the page) and Realize (lower right corner).

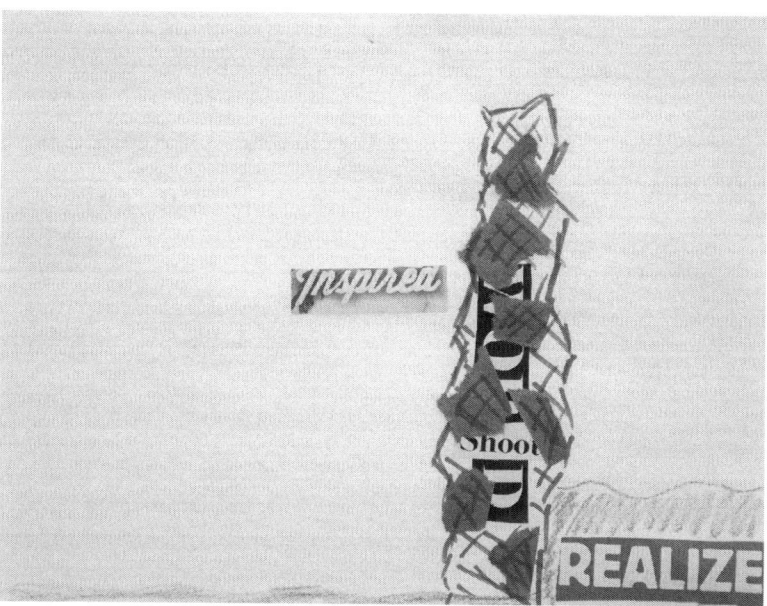

Figure 6.1 The Word

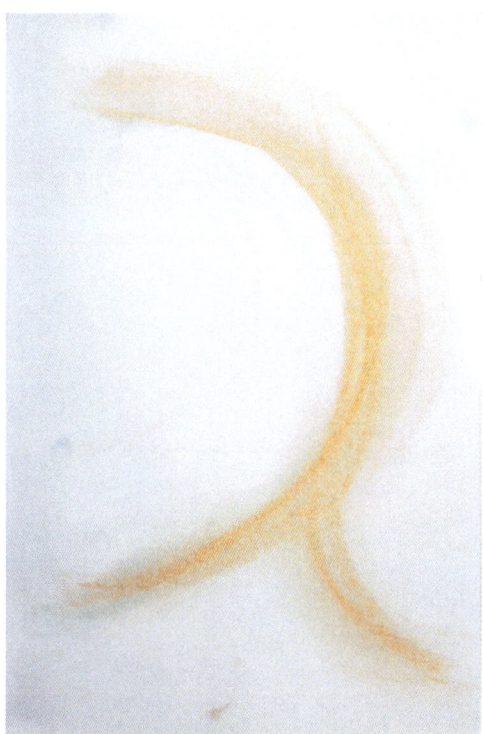

Figure 4.3 Visual Breathing

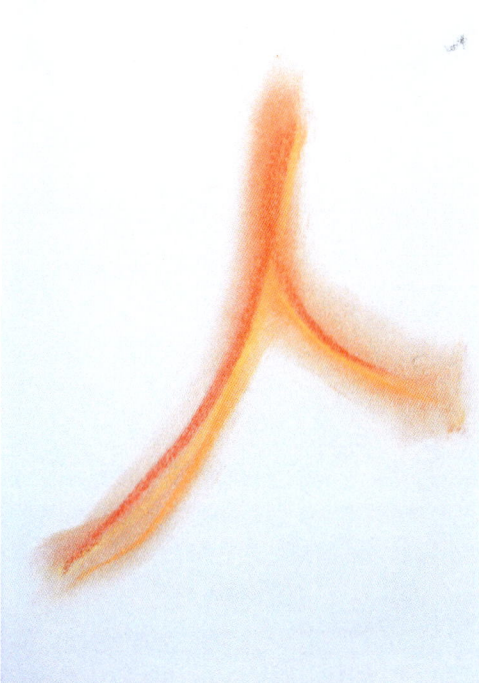

Figure 4.4 Visual Breathing

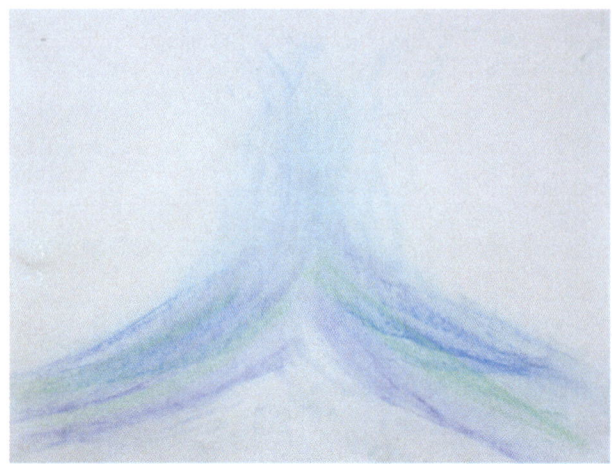

Figure 4.5 Visual Breathing

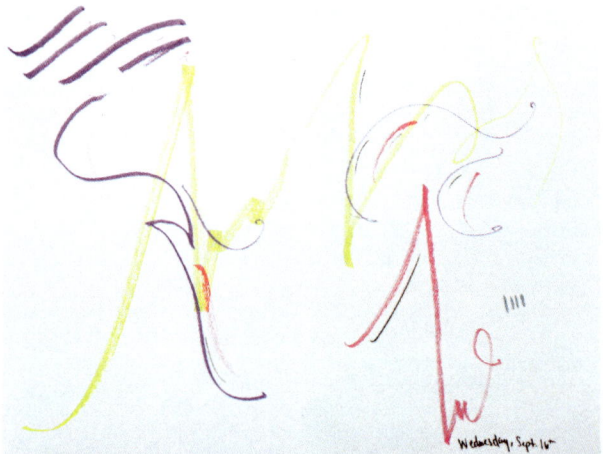

Figure 4.6 Visual Breathing

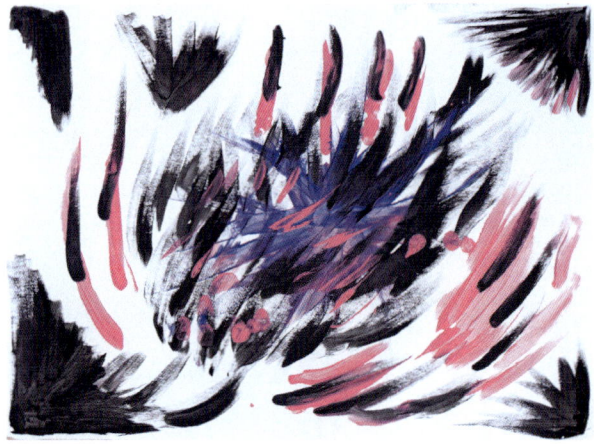

Figure 5.1 Expressive Drawings: Mind States—Mood States (Mad)

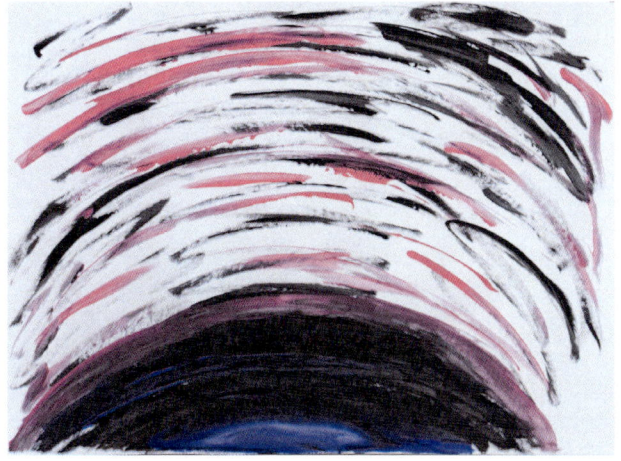

Figure 5.2 Expressive Drawings: Mind States—Mood States (Sad)

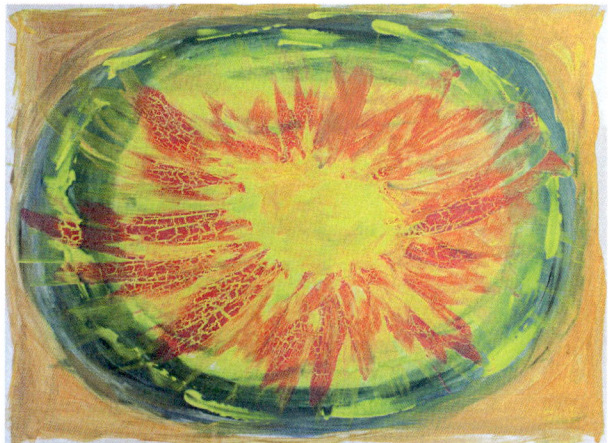

Figure 5.3 Expressive Drawings: Mind States—Mood States (Glad)

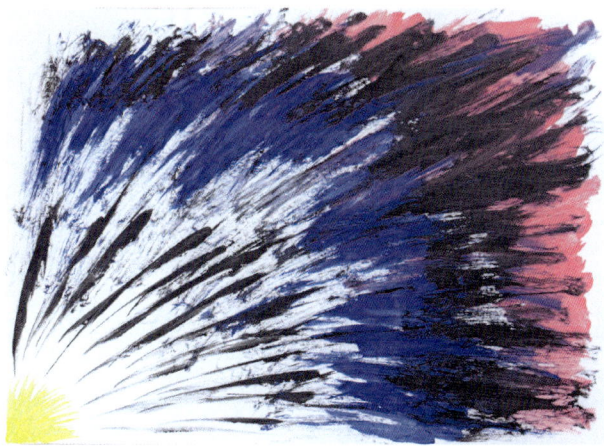

Figure 5.4 Expressive Drawings: Mind States—Mood States (Scared)

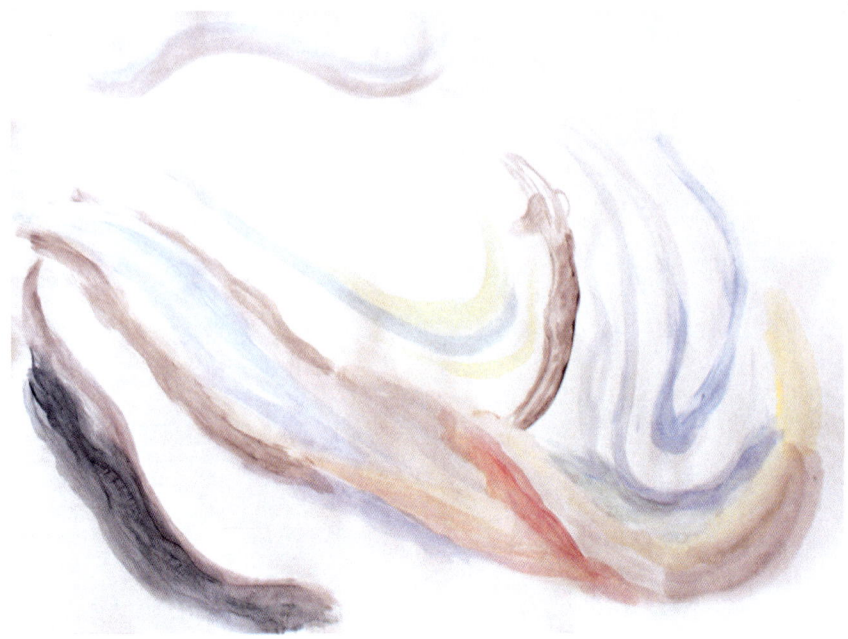

Figure 5.7 How I See Myself

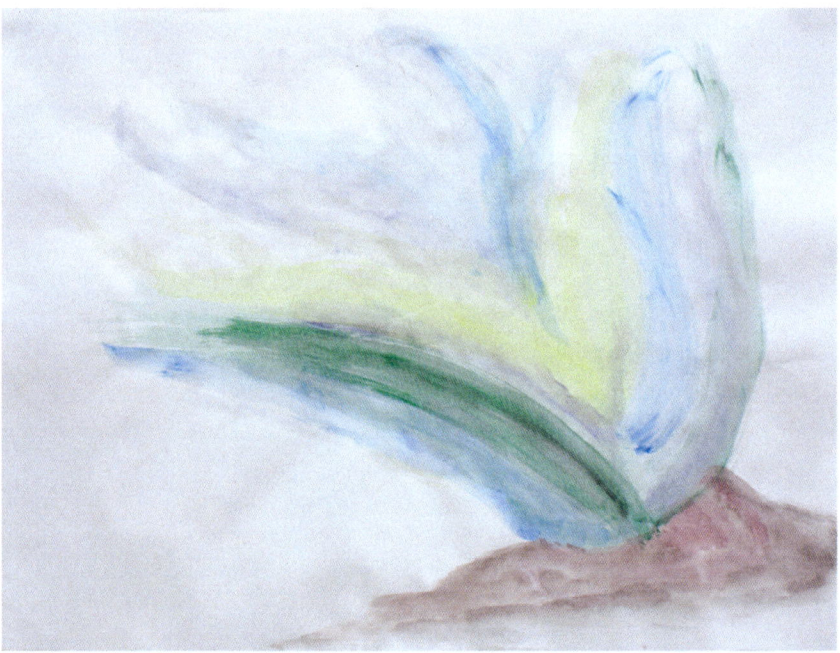

Figure 5.8 How Others See Me

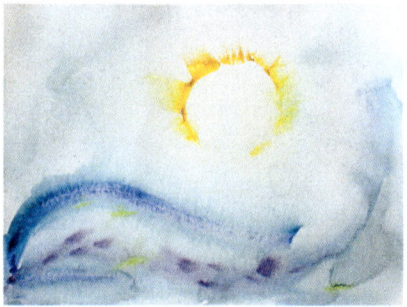

Figure 5.12 Changing Points of View 1 (Painting 1)

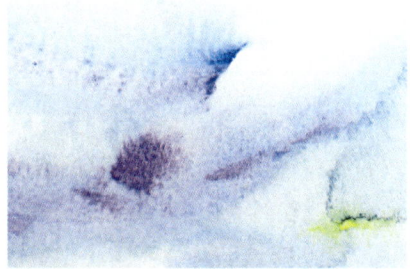

Figure 5.13 Changing Points of View 1 (Close-up)

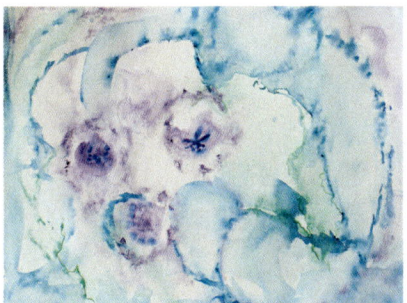

Figure 5.14 Changing Points of View 1 (Painting 2)

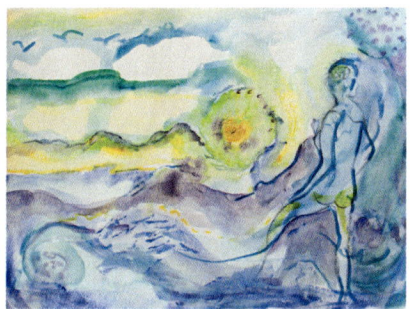

Figure 5.15 Changing Points of View 1 (Painting 3)

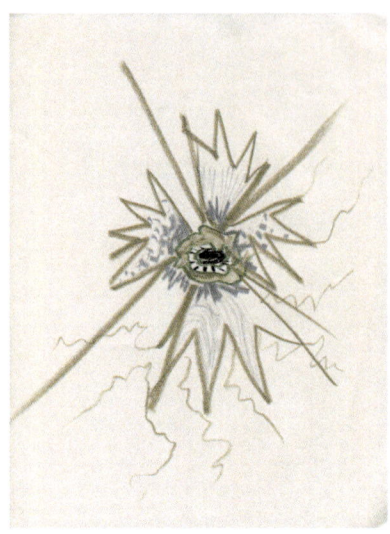

Figure 5.16 Images of Pain and Healing (Image of Pain)

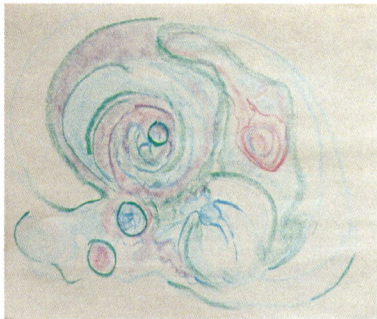

Figure 5.17 Images of Pain and Healing (Image of Healing)

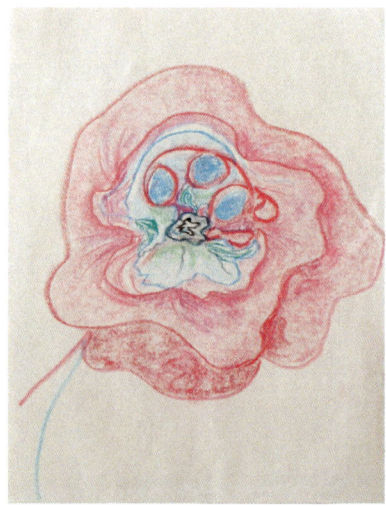

Figure 5.18 Images of Pain and Healing (Image of Healing Integrating with Pain)

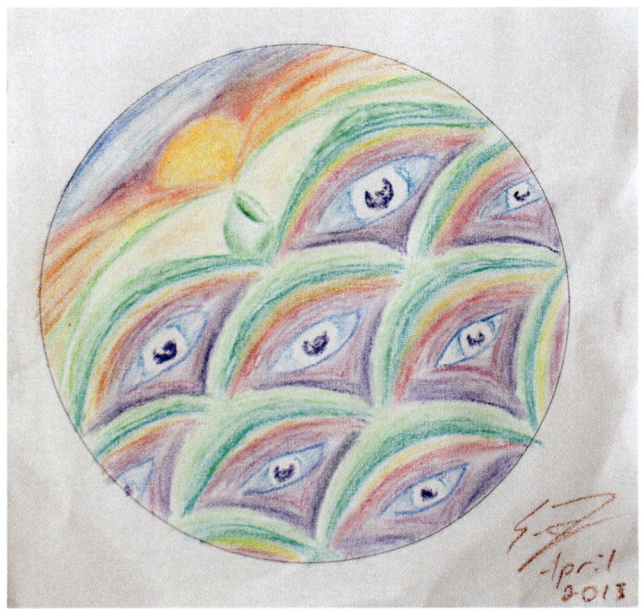

Figure 5.19 Mandala, the Great Round

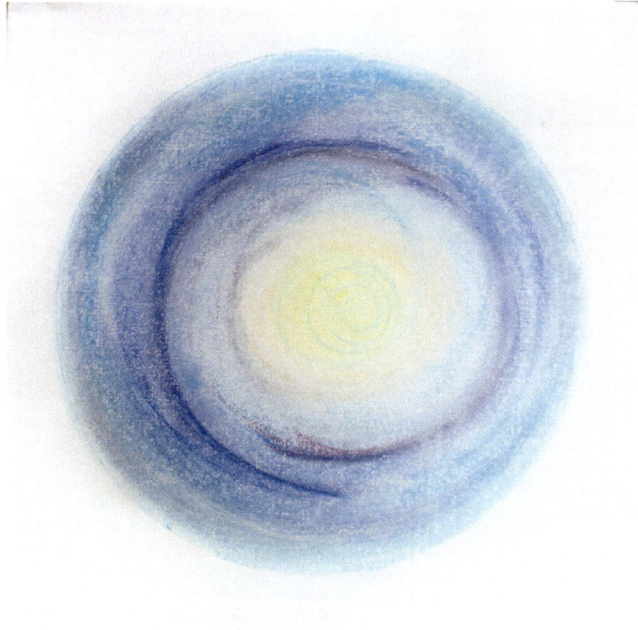

Figure 5.20 Mandala, the Great Round

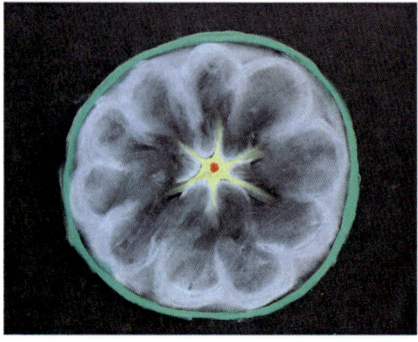

Figure 5.21 Mandala, the Great Round

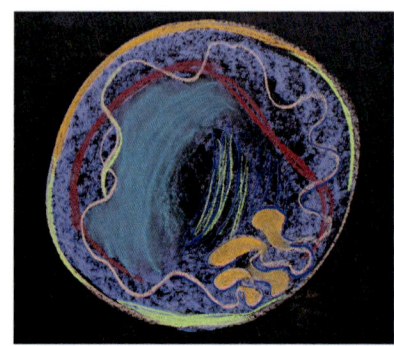

Figure 5.22 Mandala, the Great Round

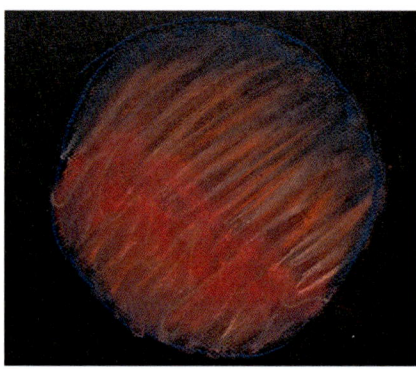

Figure 5.23 Mandala, the Great Round

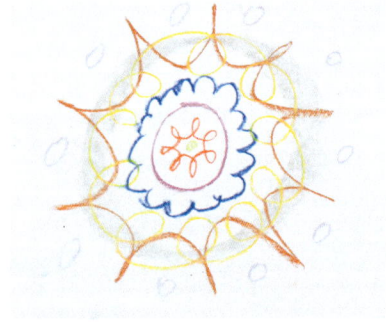

Figure 5.24 Mandala, the Great Round

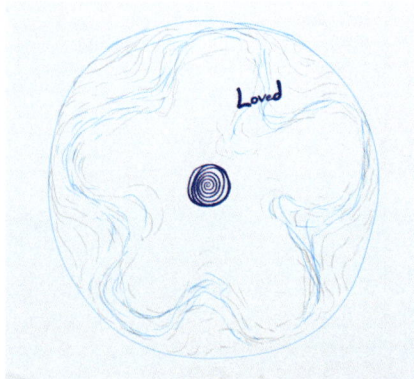

Figure 5.25 Mandala, the Great Round

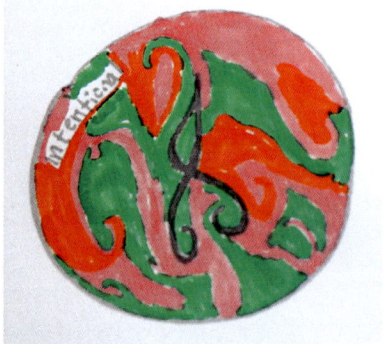

Figure 5.26 Mandala, the Great Round

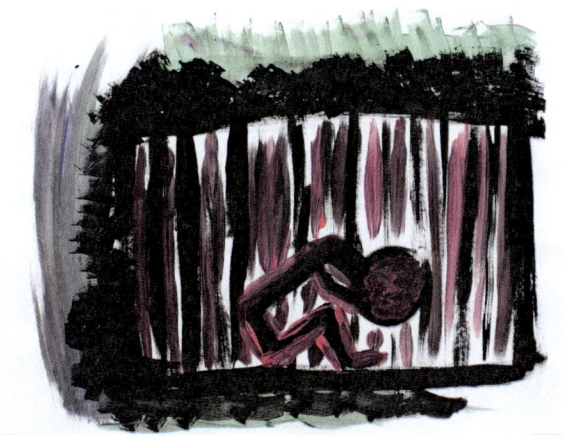

Figure 6.2 Changing Points of View 2 (Painting 1)

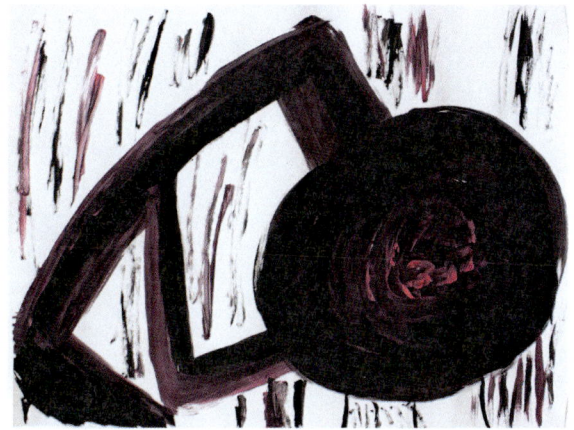

Figure 6.3 Changing Points of View 2 (Enlarge a Section)

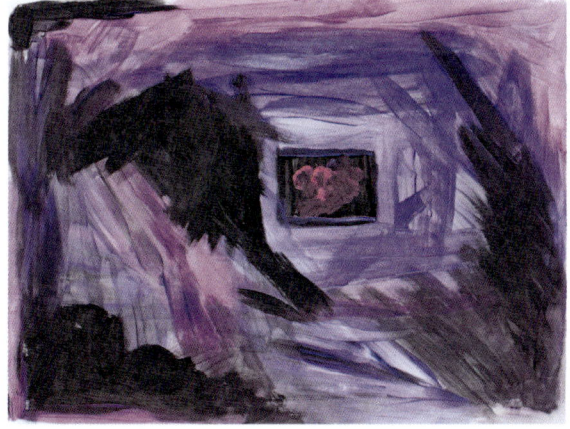

Figure 6.4 Changing Points of View 2 (Painting 3)

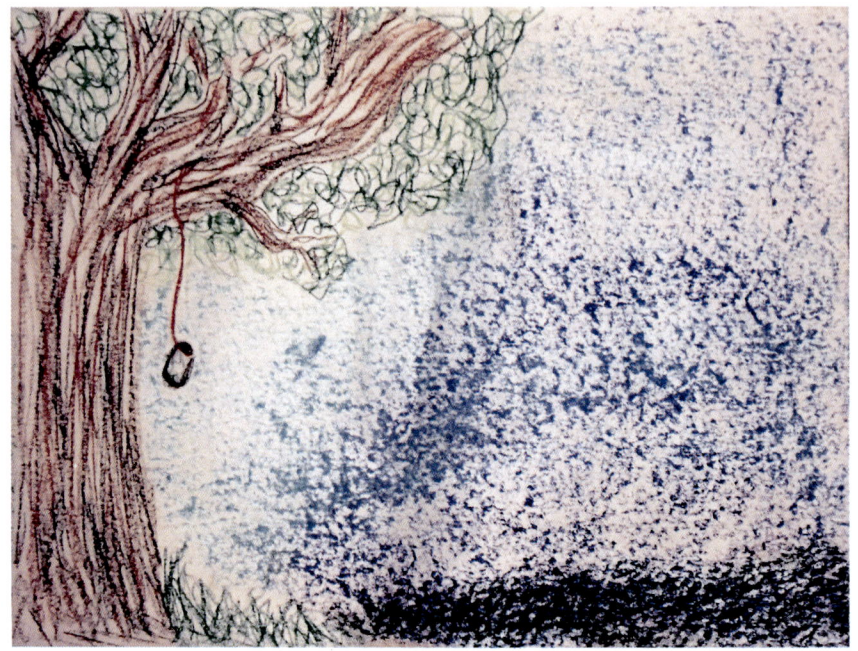

Figure 6.5 Guided Imagery—The Source

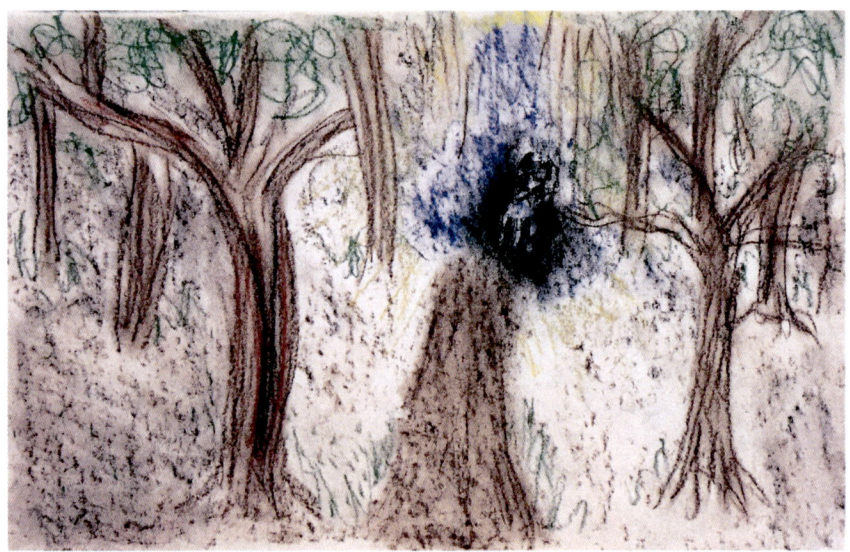

Figure 6.6 Guided Imagery— The Source

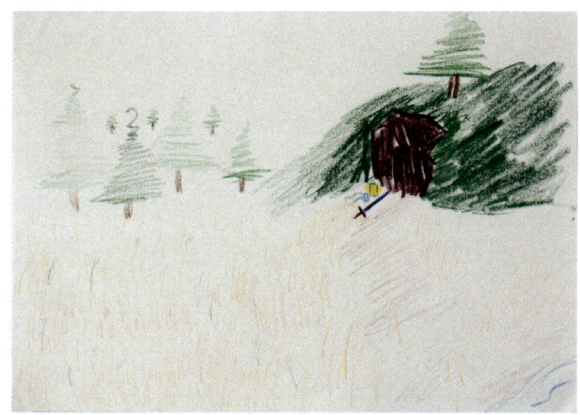

Figure 6.10 Guided Imagery—The Cave

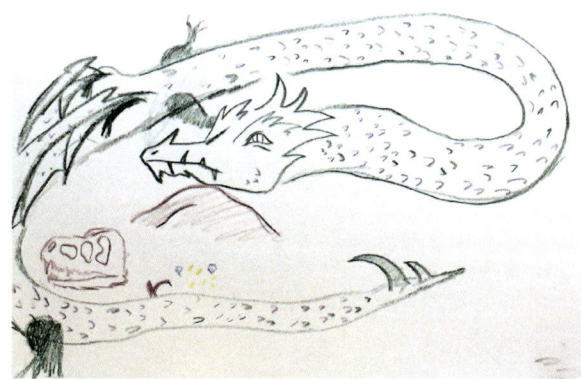

Figure 6.11 Guided Imagery—The Cave

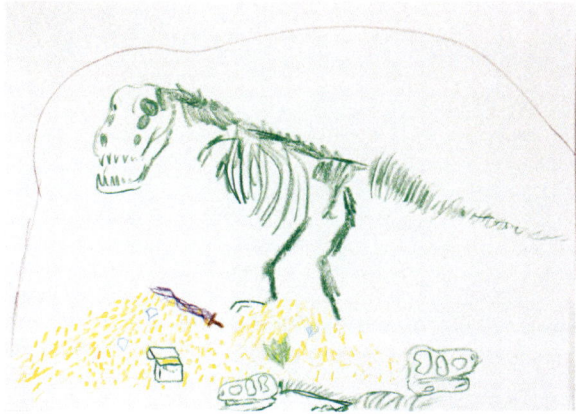

Figure 6.12 Guided Imagery—The Cave

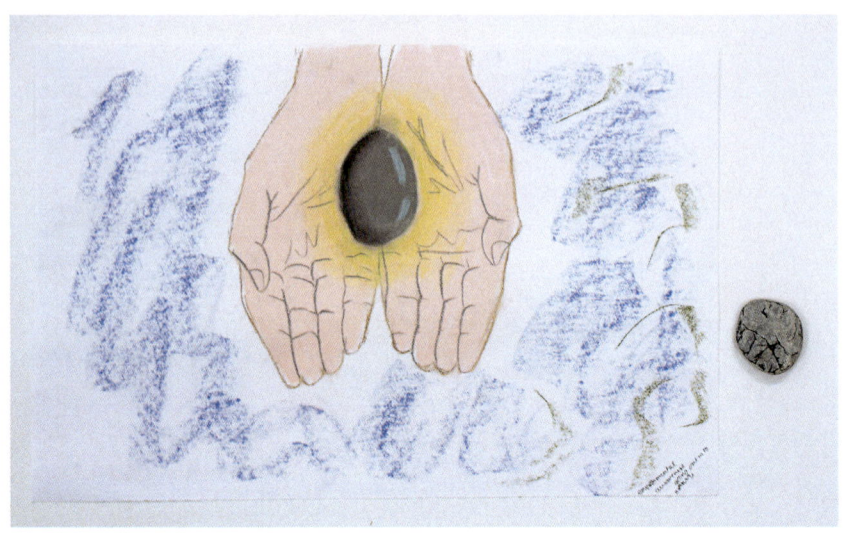

Figure 6.13 Environmental Awareness

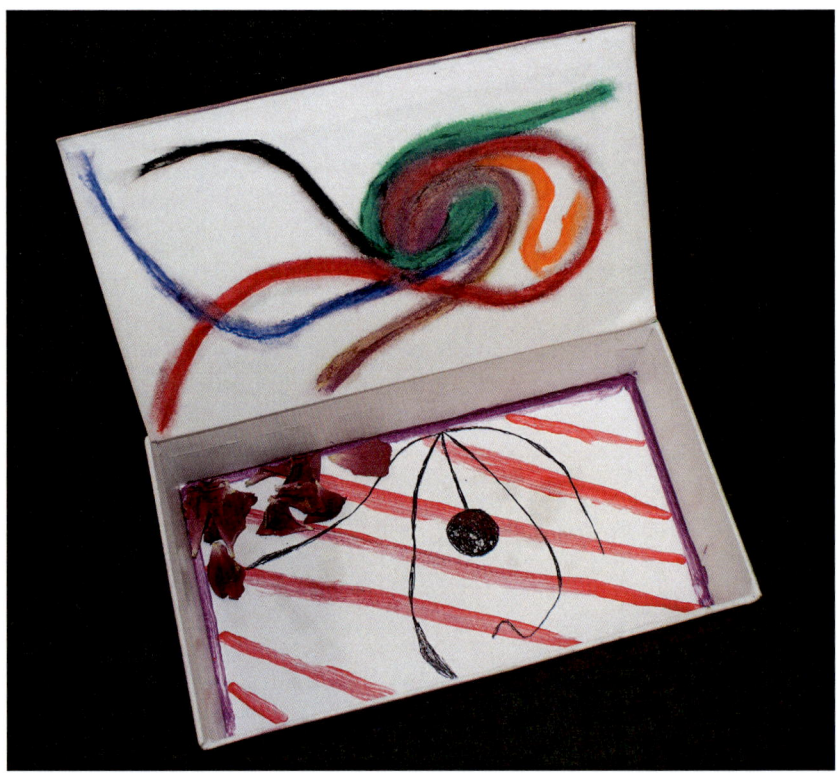

Figure 6.15 Box Self (Inner/Outer Self)

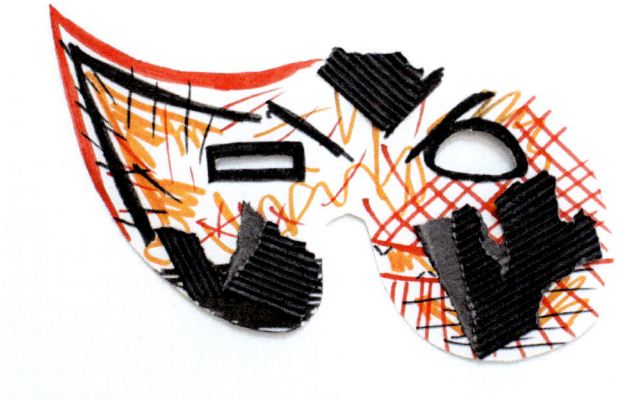

Figure 6.20 Persona Masks

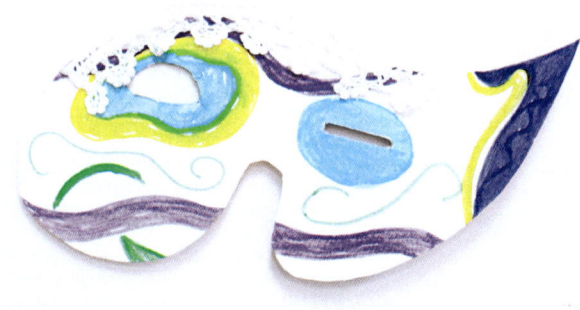

Figure 6.21 Persona Masks

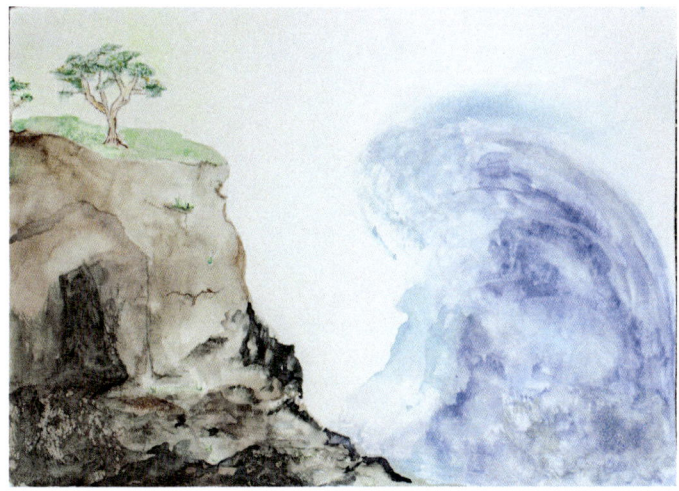

Figure 6.22 Battle Drawing

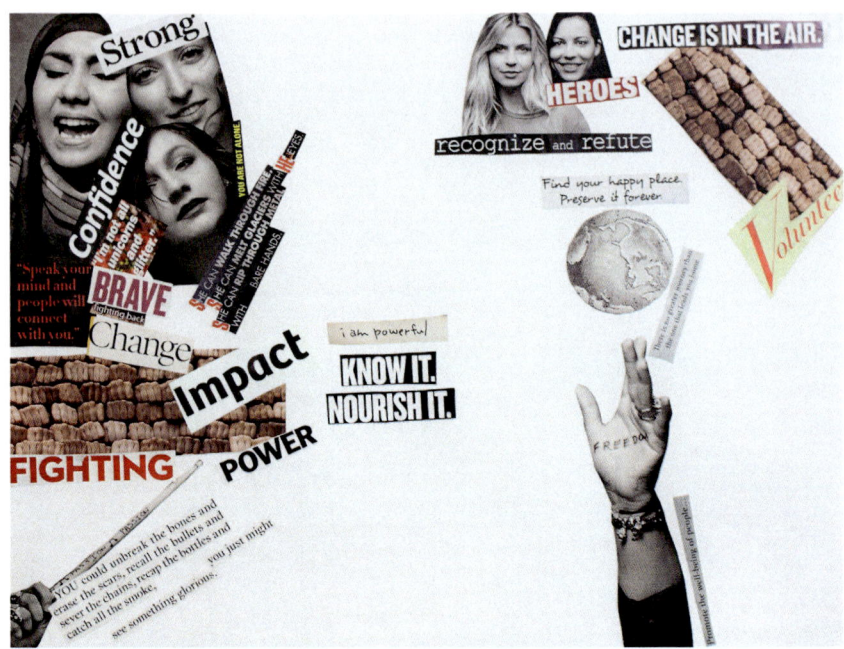

Figure 6.23 Powerful and Powerless Collage (Powerful)

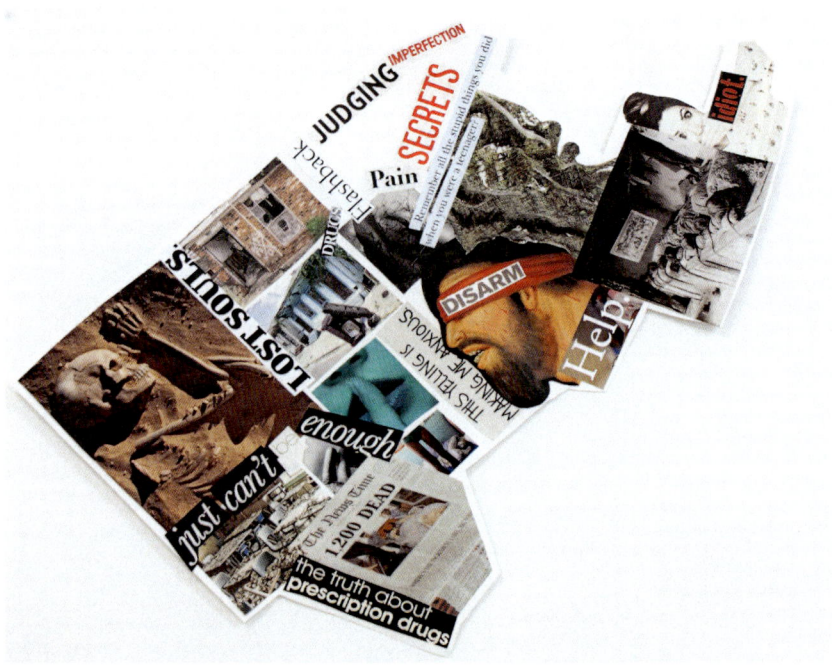

Figure 6.24 Powerful and Powerless Collage (Powerless)

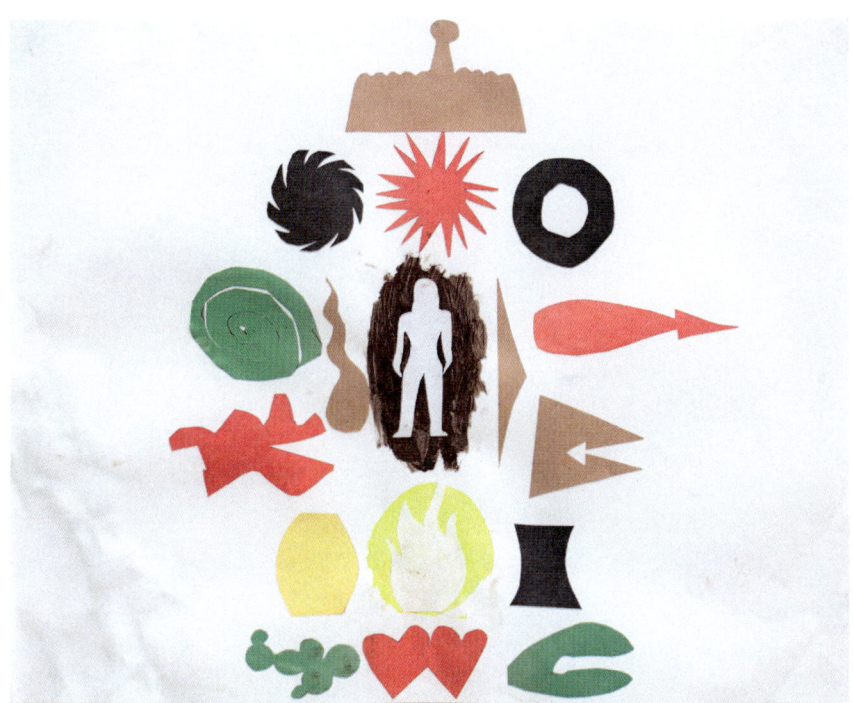

Figure 6.25 Rhyne's Problem-Solving Collage

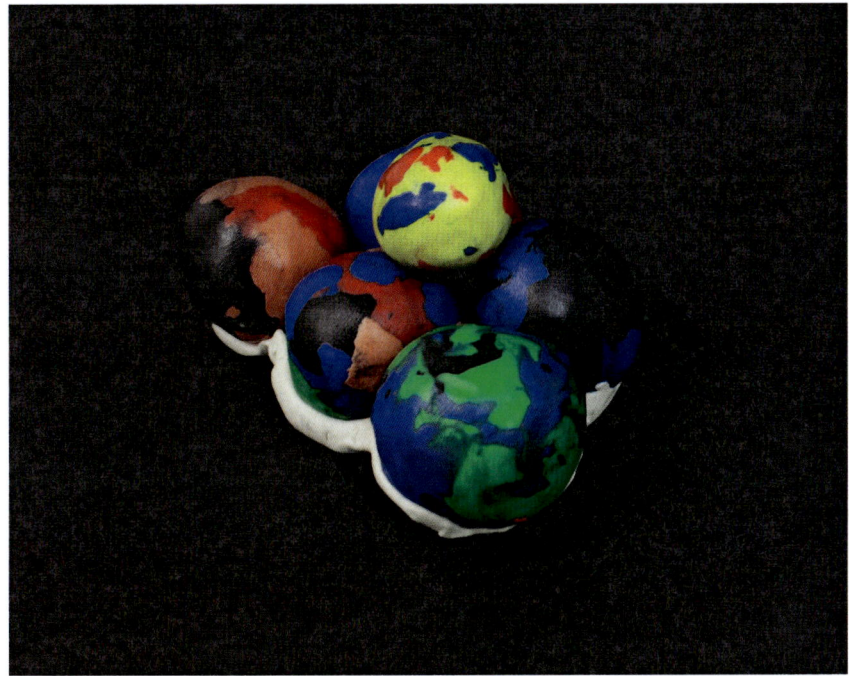

Figure 6.26 Family Sculpture

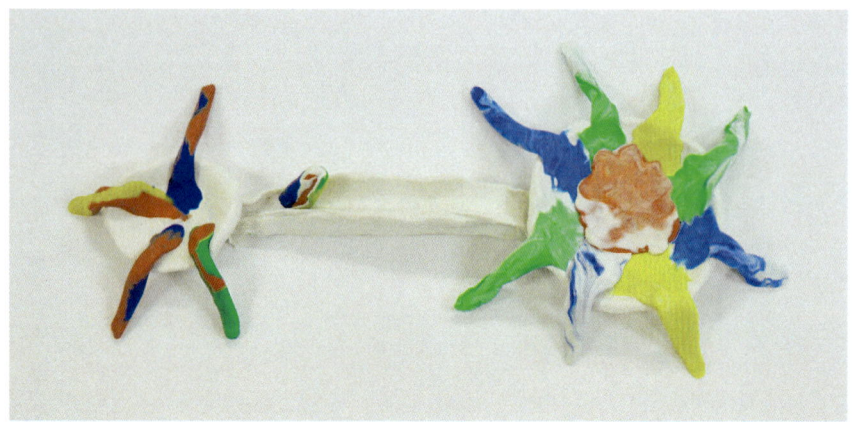

Figure 6.29 The Bridge (Bridge the Opposites)

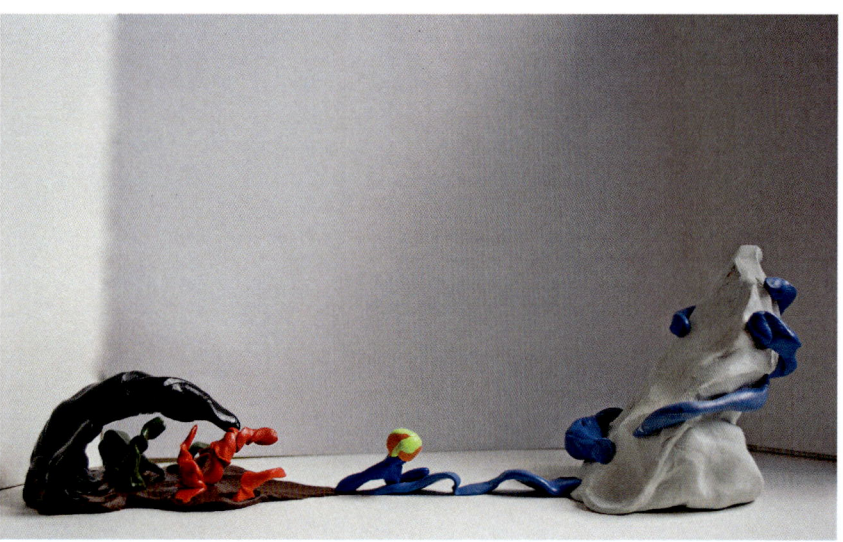

Figure 6.30 The Bridge (Bridge the Opposites)

Personal Comments—21-Year-Old Female
Undergraduate Student of Professor Kagin

I assigned meanings to each of my words (inspired, realize, world, and shoot). "Inspired" was how I see myself. "Realize" meant I want to be a person who realizes and achieves their full potential, and "World/Shoot" were clumped together as negative things holding me back from realizing my full potential. I turned the negative words into a wall between inspired and realized.

This exercise forced me to make choices that I didn't have much to say in, but also had some degree of control about my perspective on them. Like many life choices, I have to play with the cards I'm given and make the most of it. If it turns out well, that's great but can't be expected.

This made me aware of how little control I have over certain things I'm given in life (words) but also made me aware of how much control I still have over what I do with those words. Even things that don't make sense or seem valuable to begin with can be used towards a good end.

This project contains my beliefs about where I am, where I want to be, what's stopping me, and my perspective about all of it. It contains keys to awareness about how I can and do make life choices.

This forced me to see words not so much for what they are, but for whatever meaning I assigned to them. Instead of just seeing them at face value, I gave them a context in which to be seen.

Therapeutic Transition

It is notable that the tower-like figure appears to be pushing or blocking the word "realize." We would suggest she do another drawing or painting and change the position and perhaps size of the barrier, exploring the potential that is being blocked.

Creativity Activation

The application of meaning onto randomly received words forces the client to engage in a cognitive way. The creativity begins when the free association is made and then is translated into problem solving.

Adaptation

Rather than choosing the words randomly, clients could be asked to find four words in magazines or even from piles of pictures, making conscious decisions. They would then follow the steps as listed with these chosen words. The meaning would still then need to be applied from the choices they made, but they would have more of a sense of control over the words they had to use. This change could elicit even stronger responses, as clients would have to relate to choices and reactions in a new way.

Initiative Thirteen—Changing Points of View 2

ETC—Cognitive/Symbolic (C/S)
MDV—High Complexity Structured Fluid (HCSF)

Changing the words in the directive (Chapter 5) and focusing more on the cognitive symbolic can elicit significantly different responses in a client. It is the clinician's role to understand when and how an adaptation should be implemented in order to serve a client best. The following images and reflections are an example of how an adaptation to this directive was used to address a particular problem the client was having.

Materials

Tempera paint, variety of brushes to choose, 18 × 24 paper (three sheets), water, and paper towels

Directives

1. Identify a problem or challenge you are facing. It could be as minimal as a term paper that you have to write or as significant as a relationship that is struggling.
2. Paint the problem.
3. Look at the painting of your problem and take note of what you depicted and how you depicted it.
4. Enlarge a part of the problem, considering just the visuals from the first painting.
5. Finally, paint the problem smaller on the next page.
6. Look at the three paintings of your problem and examine the choices you made in each transition.
7. Process with the images.

Rationale

This initiative and its directives allow the client to explore a problem by creating a visual for it, enlarging it and then seeing it smaller as well. Theses changing perspectives, especially the minimization of the image, allow the client to see the problem on a scale that is manageable. The task of enlarging only a section forces the clients to identify visually which section they react to most strongly or see as most important. Identifying what that section represents in a larger context can often offer insights into what the real challenge is within a problem. Furthermore, the minimization of the entire issue following this discovery allows for a starting point to move forward in addressing the problem in smaller, more tangible sections: emotion, antagonist, circumstances, environment, external pressures, and so on.

Figures 6.2, 6.3, and 6.4 are the three paintings for this initiative. Figure 6.2 is a representation of a figure seated with the head bent over

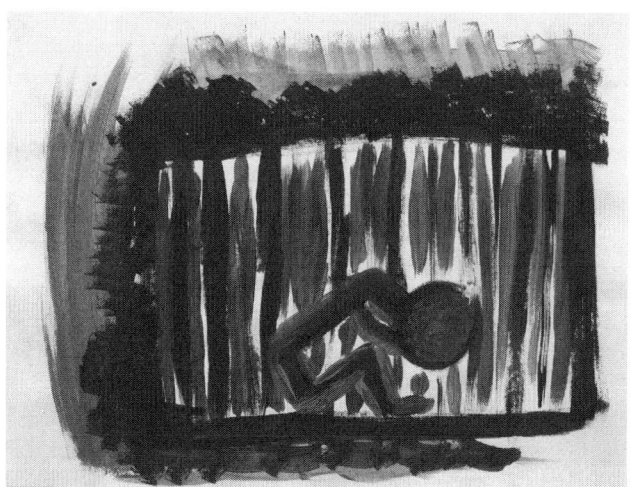

Figure 6.2 Changing Points of View 2 (Painting 1)

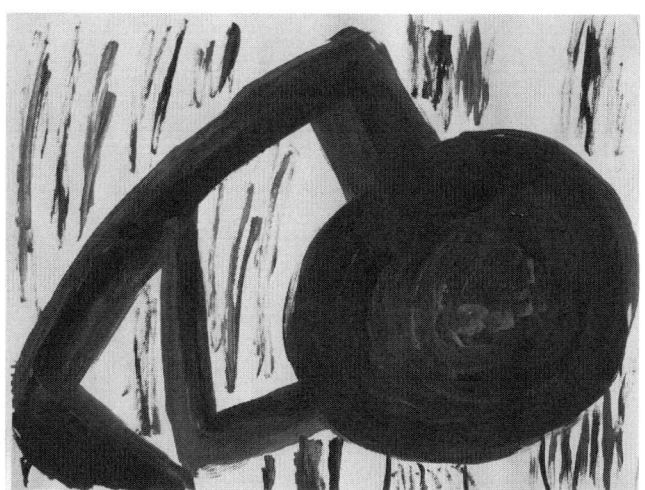

Figure 6.3 Changing Points of View 2 (Enlarge a Section)

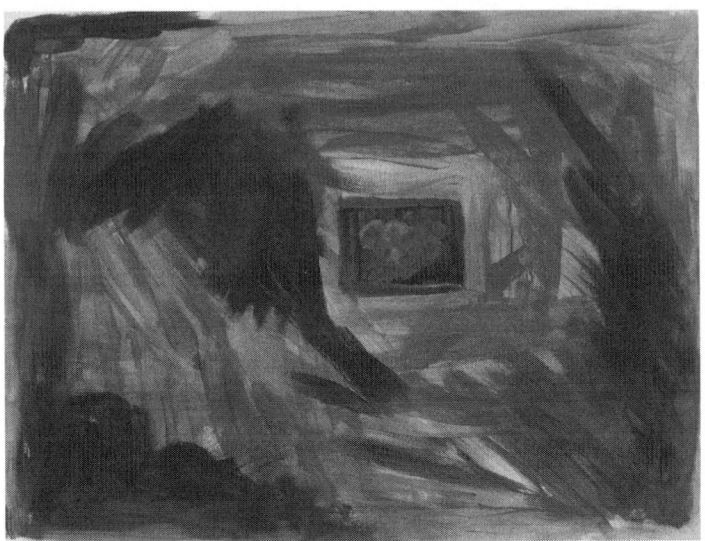

Figure 6.4 Changing Points of View 2 (Painting 3)

the knees. There is a figure in black and red in a black and red box that looks like a cage. Green paint is both under and over the lines forming the top and bottom of the box.

Figure 6.3 is the painting of the area of painting 1 (Figure 6.2) that has been enlarged. It features a large black and red circle connected to two angular lines. It is an enlargement of the figure from painting 1 (Figure 6.2).

Figure 6.4 shows the third painting in the three-part series for Changing Point of View 2. There is a small black box with red inside surrounded by violet and blue paint and large black shapes. The page is fully painted in this painting.

Personal Comments—21-Year-Old Female Undergraduate Student of Professor Kagin

This was one of the most powerful exercises for me. When we were asked to think of a problem and identify it I was a little scared because I knew what my biggest problem was, and I knew this problem had reached the point where it can no longer be avoided. The problem I chose is the emotion, anger, and identity struggles related to being sexually abused by my cousin when I was 17.

My first painting was an abstract human form in a cage with heavy black bars and hints of red inside the cage, with color trying to get in. This explains my overall understanding of the problem and my inability to escape it and how it overshadows the good colorful part of my life. Then we were asked to make a part of the problem bigger and the second I painted a black circle creating the head of my figure I knew what it meant and there was no turning back. This painting showed that although I know it wasn't my fault I still experience feelings that I am to blame and that I could have done something to change it. Thinking deeper these problems stem from being asked by my family over and over why I let it happen to me.

Then the final painting was to make the problem smaller and I tried really hard to minimize it but the black kept coming out and covering my bright colors. This showed me that I feel a lack of control in containing this problem because it bleeds into every part of my life.

I shared these insights with the class and felt the need to share my story with the group despite my fear of being vulnerable. I just needed to let the words out. I had constantly drained myself of the images of this trauma, but I scarcely honestly opened up about the pain and confusion and overall defeat I feel.

Therapeutic Transition

This young woman needs to see that the color in her life does not have to be overshadowed by her trauma. Although the trauma is part of her, it does not define her. We suggest she be given the Powerful/Powerless collage to enable her to focus on how the shame and anger are affecting her behavior and sense of self. The material usage of the collage moves her from the P/A to the C/S because it is a less fluid experience and she can focus on the cognitive.

Creativity Activation

The creativity level is activated in this exercise when the client is asked to enlarge a section of their original painting (problem). This taps into the creative problem solving by altering the perception of the problem.

Adaptation

See Changing Point of View 1 in Chapter 5.

Introduction to Guided Imagery

The use of guided imagery relies heavily on lowering the brain waves to a relaxed beta or theta state and allowing unconscious images to merge with limbic responses. Guided imagery is a form of focus, altering perception and mindfulness that assists the rerouting of brain synaptic patterns that may have been there since early childhood.

We have focused on archetypal symbols and experiences, in more specific cases, on trauma relief, but there are literally hundreds of scripted meditations online for health and wellness, healing, stress relief, positive thinking. As a clinician, you may select what is most pertinent to your patient. A word of advice, however, and this is true of using any of the initiatives in this book—do it yourself first! When you are relaxing your client, watch their breathing and any body movements carefully. In some cases it may be necessary to put yourself into the imagery as a supportive companion.

Initiative Fourteen—Guided Imagery—The Source

ETC—Cognitive/Symbolic (C/S)
MDV—High Complexity Structured Fluid (HCSF)

Materials

Comfortable mat or chair, three pieces watercolor paper (12 × 18), variety of brush sizes, watercolor, tempera or acrylic, or pastels. In some cases, you may substitute watercolor markers or colored pencils to give the person more control depicting their journey.

Directives

1. Conduct breathing relaxation initiative in a low-light, quiet environment.
2. When person is in a very relaxed state, softly direct as follows:
   You are lying in softness, much like a cloud embracing you. You trust this cloud and allow it to help you travel.
   The cloud is slowly lifting you, swaying with a gentle breeze. You feel warm and safe.
   After a few minutes, the cloud begins to descend and places you gently into a meadow. Look around you. See the meadow and what is in it. Feel the sun: not too hot, not too cool. There is a very slight breeze. Breathe in the fragrances around you as you sit up and further observe your meadow.
   Off to your left, you see a stream. Get up and walk to the bank of the stream. Gaze at the water, its flow, its clarity. Is there anything in the stream? How do the banks look?
   Along the stream you notice a path and begin to walk it. The path follows the stream, both always in your sight. As you walk your path, you notice it has an incline and appears to be getting steeper. You continue walking.
   Ahead of you is an object obstructing your path. Go to this object. Contemplate it. How do you get to the other side to continue along the path?
   After you have overcome your obstacle, you notice that your walk has become a climb. It is more difficult and becoming quite steep.
   Up ahead is the top of your journey. Finish your climb.

Look around you, and you will see the source of your stream. Sit beside it and rest after a job well done.

Next to you is a vessel. Pick it up. Observe it, feel it and hold it up to the sunlight.

Now lower your vessel into the source, fill it, and take a drink. See the peacefulness and beauty around you and know that at any time, you may return to this place, as it belongs only to you.

Refill the vessel, stand and look around your source, then head back down the path, carrying the vessel with you.

Does the path seem different on the way down and back? Does the stream look or feel different on the way down and back? Your obstacle is no longer a challenge, and you easily traverse the path back to your meadow.

As you look up ahead of you, see someone waiting there for you.

Go to that person and offer a drink from your vessel. You each have something to say to the other before you leave.

Now put the vessel on the ground and turn, heading back to your cloud-filled landing place. Relax deeply into the cloud as it lifts you gently and carries you back to this room. Slowly become aware of your body, and when you are ready, open your eyes and return to this room.

3. Paint three pictures of your journey: your meadow, your source, and your vessel, all on separate pieces of paper. Remember that the visual image is difficult to translate into paint pigment and paper, so be patient.
4. If you feel there are other symbols that had even more meaning to you, draw or paint those as well on separate pieces of paper.

Rationale

There are many very important and powerful symbols in the source. We again refer you to the *Book of Symbols*, edited by Ami Ronnberg and Kathleen Martin and overseen by the Jung Foundation and Archive for Research in Archetypal Symbolism.

Processing the three paintings is done by informing the client of the possible meaning of each of the symbols. If these meanings seem significant to that person, then help apply them to their life, quest, conflict, or whatever has brought the person to therapy.

As a group exercise, divide into pairs and let each share their discoveries.

Figures 6.5 and 6.6 correspond to this initiative. They show an image of a large tree on the left of the page with a jar hanging from the branch (Figure 6.5) and a forest with a path in the center and a form in black and blue at the end (Figure 6.6).

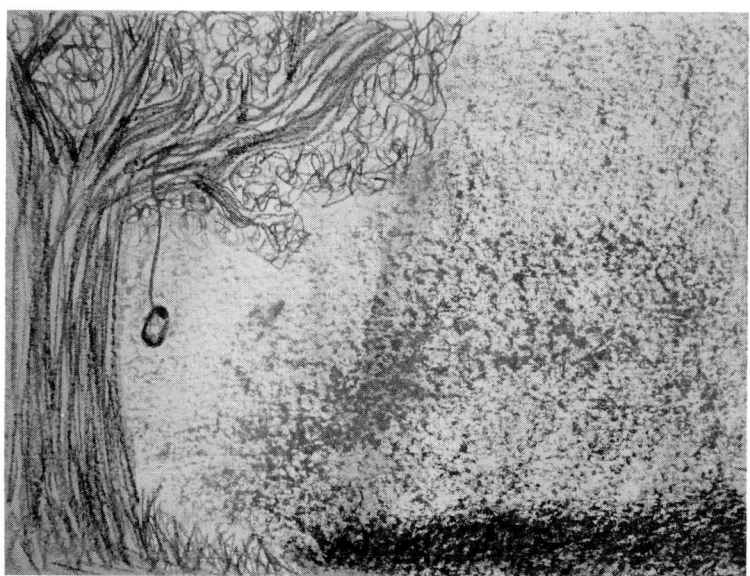

Figure 6.5 Guided Imagery—The Source

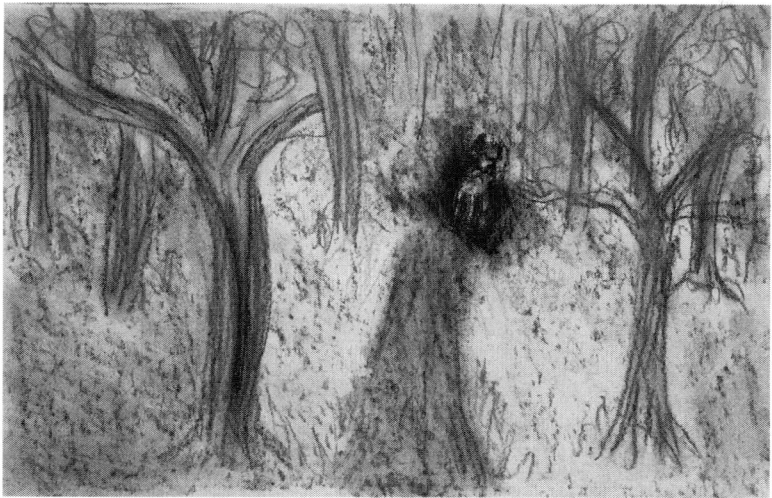

Figure 6.6 Guided Imagery—The Source

Personal Comments—Author Two, Christa Kagin, When She Was in Graduate School

This was not uplifting for me, but rather painful. My encounter was with my dog who had died in October. The place was comforting, my grandpa's land where Ty (my dog) is buried and the source was the pond.

The vessel was a mason jar that Papa uses to drink his tea. I had a new puppy, Boomer, and this brought up many fears of loss beyond those associated with Ty, and the heartache of losing my friend. It was metaphorical for loss. I have been no stranger to grief in my life. I really needed to draw the encounter. Later I realized that the mason jar was a feminine component and it was reminiscent of canning, sustenance, nurturance, strength, birth and history.

I felt as if I was drinking from my family, my strength of support, and going to safety, Papa's place. In dissecting each part I found comfort.

As we are writing this book years later and I look at these images I am having a very poignant experience as both my grandfather and Boomer have died.

The family sold my grandfather's farm and land this year and I have grieved that more than I ever realized I would. So now as I look at this image of the mason jar hanging in a tree, to be discovered along a journey, it is comforting to think that even though Papa and the farm are no longer with me, I will still be renewed and refreshed from what they have left behind in my heart. I was also facing physical challenges at that time and was not emotionally addressing it. My grief was represented in my fear of my own health and being incapacitated.

It is relevant to mention here that the power of the image is not only healing and insightful at the time of creation, but what we understand about the containment abilities of art is also evident in this vignette, as a return to the image years later is still cathartic and healing.

Therapeutic Transition

It would have been appropriate to explore the grief further. Use of a lifeline would be beneficial, as many of the memories of childhood were related to her grandfather and that farm.

Creativity Activation

Creativity is first initiated when visualization begins in the imagination during guided imagery as spoken by the therapist. This is further realized when the images are translated from the mind to the page. Media will also impact the creativity as the individual resonates with its property.

Adaptations

Adaptations relate to what you focus on and what you extract as the symbols for representation. These could vary by client but should be carefully considered, as changes can certainly elicit different responses.

Initiative Fifteen—Guided Imagery—The Dwelling

ETC—Cognitive/Symbolic (C/S)
MDV—High Complexity Structured Fluid (HCSF)

Materials

Comfortable mat or chair, three pieces watercolor paper (12 × 18), variety of brush sizes, watercolor, tempera or acrylic, or pastels. In some cases, you may substitute watercolor markers or colored pencils to give the person more control depicting their journey.

Directives

1. Conduct breathing relaxation initiative in a low-light, quiet environment.
2. Use the breathing initiative until the person becomes totally relaxed, with eyes closed. The room should be quiet and the light low. When person is in a very relaxed state, softly direct as follows:

    Today you will be going for a walk. You will begin in a meadow. The sun is shining on you, and it is the perfect temperature outside. There is a soft breeze.

    Prepare yourself to take a walk, knowing that you will be climbing, because in the distance you can see a small mountain. What will you take with you? Lift your pack and put it on. Stand in the meadow, take a deep breath, feel the sun warm on your face, and begin on this journey. As you walk, take in the sounds around you. Look at the clear blue sky.

    After some time of walking, you come to the base of the small mountain, and you decide to keep walking, climbing up. There is a path you are traveling along, indicating that others have walked here as well. As you keep walking, you begin to feel the incline increasing. Still, you are energized and keep going. There are many trees along the path, but you can easily maneuver the path. After a short time, you encounter an obstacle, something on the path before you. You must decide what to do. How will you get past this obstacle?

    Once you have solved moving past the obstacle, you continue on your path, winding and climbing up. Again, there is something obstructing the clearing of your path. This time, it is more challenging to traverse, but you persevere because you have come so far and you want to reach the top. Just around the small bend, you notice the path continues on in one direction, but there is a slight clearing that goes straight, and you could change your route. Do you take this other path?

Climbing and hiking on, you feel good about your ability to get beyond the obstacles in your way, and you are enjoying the strength you feel as you climb and travel to the top, which you have almost reached. Just a short distance ahead, you see the sun shining brightly and an opening in the trees where the path seems to end. You have nearly reached the top! As you walk through the last trees, a clearing opens before you, a plateau on the top of the mountain. Before you is a meadow similar to the one you began from, but this one is at the top of the mountain, where you can see far off in the distance. As you stand and look around, your eye catches sight of a dwelling before you. You begin to walk toward it. As you approach, you can see that it looks as if no one is around, but others have been here. Will you look inside? Knock on the door? Walk around it? What do you find? Spend some time here. Enjoy this place and, after a while, prepare to return to the meadow.

The walk down the mountain is good, and you feel peaceful and happy. This has been an amazing journey today. As you end your walk and approach the meadow again, turn and look back. *You* climbed that mountain today and moved past obstacles. It has been a good day.

3. Draw or paint three images, each on a separate piece of paper: The items packed for the journey, the obstacle you encountered, and the dwelling at the top of the mountain.
4. Process by discussing the experience, the images created, and the symbolic meaning of each.

Rationale

The symbolic choices for clients as they experience the guided imagery and make decisions about objects, challenges, and encounters can provide insightful gains. Often when a client responds positively to guided imagery, therapists may use a series of scripts to explore responses and variations from one to the other. Commonly used symbols the client or student uses on this journey are the meadow (which we define as a place of homeostasis), tools for survival (such as food and water) or comfort, or symbolic challenges such as a backpack, which may represent the maternal feminine responsibility and burdens associated with it. Specific symbols can be researched by the client and therapist or teacher.

Figures 6.7, 6.8, and 6.9 show the drawing from this Initiative. Figure 6.7 shows the objects taken on the journey: camera, water

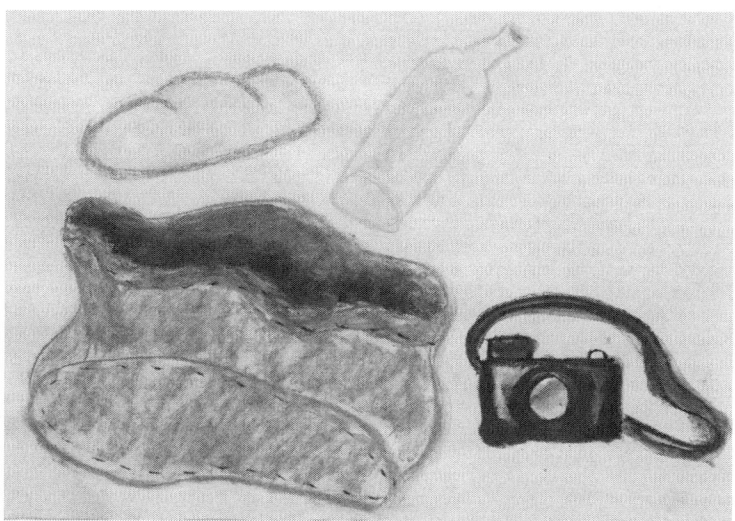

Figure 6.7 Guided Imagery—Dwelling

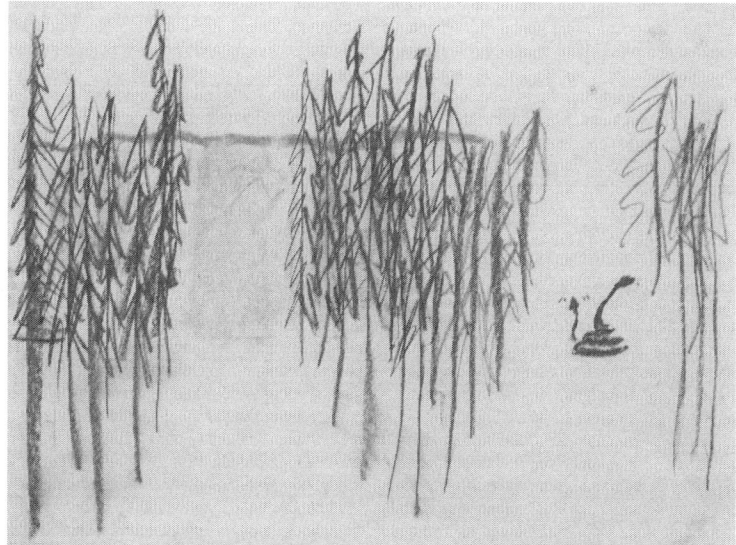

Figure 6.8 Guided Imagery—Dwelling

Figure 6.9 Guided Imagery—Dwelling

bottle, bread, and bag. Figure 6.8 is a representation of the forest and the obstacles encountered: a cliff and a snake. Figure 6.9 is a drawing of the dwelling found at the top of the mountain. It depicts the dwelling, the stream of water, a wheel, and a suggestion of trees in the background. Coming out of the chimney are purple and yellow stars.

Personal Comments—20-Year-Old Female Undergraduate Student of Professor Kagin

In this exercise, I packed very practically. I packed some bread in case I became hungry on my journey, water in case I became thirsty, an oversized bag to put the things in in case I found things along my journey that I wanted to keep, and a camera in case there were sights or moments I wanted to remember.

These obstacles were somewhat personal, but not deeply. I have an unreasonable fear of snakes so naturally that was one of my obstacles, I believe what happened in my story is that I picked it up with a long stick and threw it into the woods. The other obstacle was a cliff that was impossible to scale, and looked hopeless and impossible, so I climbed a tree and hopped onto the top of the cliff instead.

This was a small dwelling I came upon before I reached my final destination. There was a river that had a wheel in it, (the river eventually gave way to a waterfall going off the edge of a cliff at the final destination) and there were sparkles coming out of the chimney representing a wizard that lived inside the cabin.

I never actually made it to the top of the mountain, though that was my original goal when I was standing in the field looking at my oncoming journey. Instead, there was a fork in the road, one that led to my original destination and one that was unknown. I chose the unknown destination and it turned out much more beautiful than just the peak of the mountain, because I ended up on the side of the mountain, looking at the world through a misty waterfall and a vibrant forest beneath me.

Overall the journey was enjoyable, exciting, and at the end of it I had a sense of peace from the choices I had made along the way.

Therapeutic Transition

Not actually making it to the top of the mountain (an original goal) could be explored, and the idea of fantasy could be excavated in drawing form. Who was the wizard? What would he say or do? Was he familiar? These questions could address the possibility of flight as the student changed directions and allowed herself the option of not achieving the climax of the climb. Is this a pattern of behavior? What might happen if she persevered? What holds her back? Exploration of the roles she plays in her life and whether she is avoidant of challenge in complex or uncertain situations could help to identify a pattern of behavior and strengthen resiliency traits.

Adaptation

Omitting the bend in the path and the option for clients to change their course would address the option of not reaching the climax of the mountain. This could serve to intentionally move them on to the dwelling and the mountaintop. Conversely, it eliminates the opportunity for the client to learn about their behavioral pattern of not persevering at times. Additionally, you could lead the client into the dwelling and omit the option of entering or looking through a window. This would have to be carefully considered and be specific to each client, as it could elicit fear and anxiety.

Initiative Sixteen—Guided Imagery—The Cave

ETC—Cognitive/Symbolic (C/S)
MDV—High Complexity Structured Fluid (HCSF)

Materials

Comfortable mat or chair, three pieces watercolor paper (12 × 18), variety of brush sizes, watercolor, tempera or acrylic, or pastels. In some cases, you may substitute watercolor markers or colored pencils to give the person more control depicting their journey.

Directives

1. Conduct breathing relaxation initiative in a low-light, quiet environment.
2. Use the breathing initiative until the person becomes totally relaxed, with eyes closed. The room should be quiet and the light low. When person is in a very relaxed state, softly direct as follows:

    You are in a meadow. The sun is warm but not hot, and there is a quiet breeze. Standing in your meadow, turn slowly around and observe as many details as possible. To your right, you see the opening to what appears to be a cave. Walk toward that opening. When you get there, you peek inside. It is dark and is indeed a cave, but you do not know how large. Outside the entrance are three objects: a pouch, a lantern, and a sword. You decide which or all you wish to use to explore the cave and pick them up. Go inside the cave. The temperature is comfortable. You are not afraid. Look around you as you take each step. What do you observe? Keep walking as you go deeper into the cavern. You hear something ahead.

    Slowly moving forward, you discover a dragon. This dragon is guarding a treasure, and you realize it is your treasure. You want to see this treasure but must get around the dragon first. Remember the pouch, lantern, and sword as you contemplate the dragon. Take action and go to your treasure. What do you see? Do you wish to take it with you? When you are ready to leave, follow the path you took to the entrance. Does it look different to you? When you come to

the entrance, replace what you took with you, leaving the pouch, lantern, and sword for the next adventurer. You are back in your meadow. Lie down and slowly count to three before opening your eyes and reentering the room.
3. Paint three pictures, one on each piece of paper: cave entrance with pouch, lantern, and sword, the dragon, and the treasure.
4. Process the significance of each symbol and the journey into the cave as a whole.

Rationale

The symbols in this guided imagery are also Jungian based. The Cave, a passage between this world and the underworld, and/or the mother (womb); the Lantern, to shine, be bright, consciousness to maintain life, hope, and creativity; the Pouch, container of personal identity, psychic energy (intuition), and sexual boundaries; the Sword, the warrior; and the Treasure, fame, transcendence, goals, sometimes shame (Ronnberg and Martin, 2010). It is a more challenging journey, as entering the cave (the unconscious) can be anxiety inducing. Reassure the participant that it is safe to journey inward as you proceed.

Figures 6.10, 6.11, and 6.12 are the drawings for the Cave Initiative. Figure 6.10 shows the meadows in yellow, with the cave on the right side (deep purple) and the three objects lying (sword, bag, and lantern) at the entrance. Drawn in colored pencil, you can see the texture and pressure variations from the marks. Trees surround the entrance.

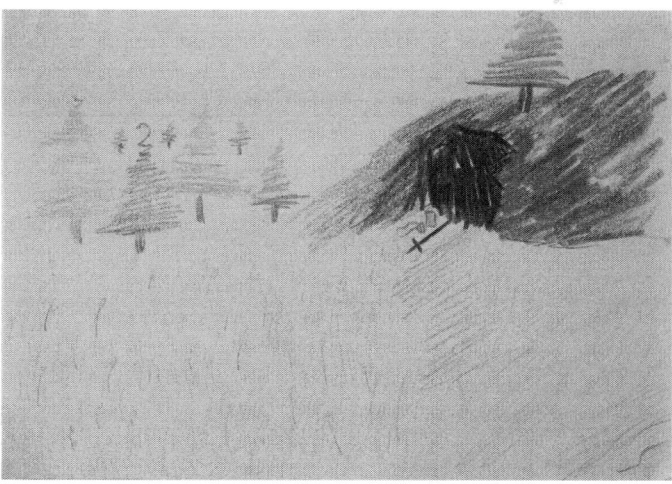

Figure 6.10 Guided Imagery—The Cave

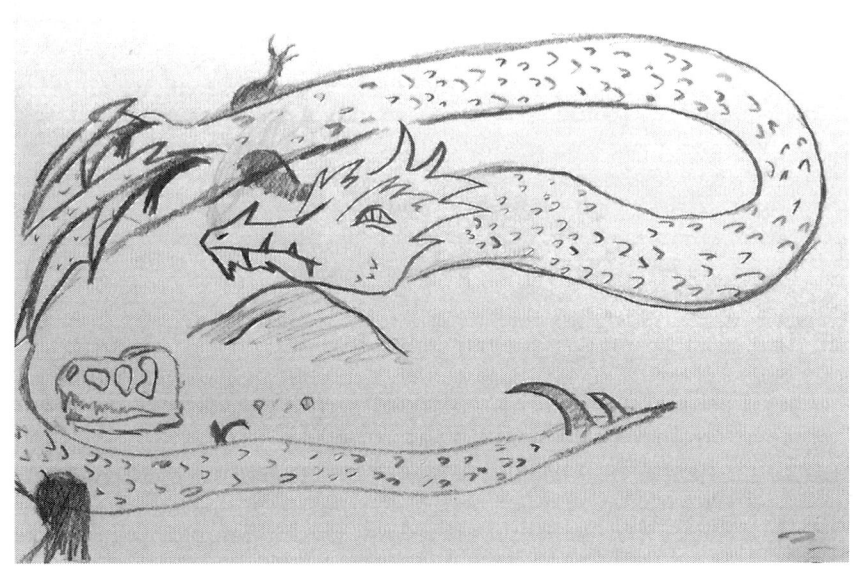

Figure 6.11 Guided Imagery—The Cave

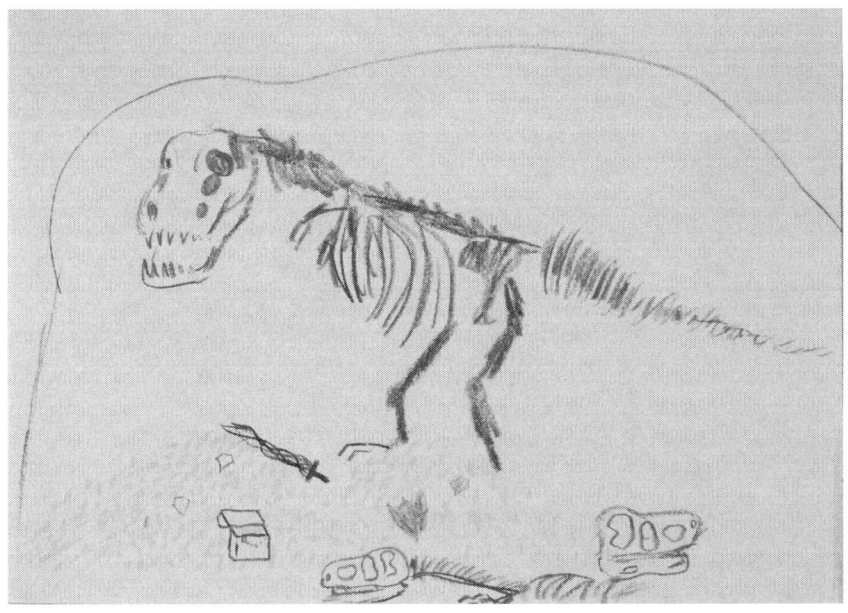

Figure 6.12 Guided Imagery—The Cave

Figure 6.11 is a drawing of the dragon in green outlines with suggested scales. Figure 6.12 is the image of the treasure found inside the cave: dinosaur skeletons, a pile of gold, and a treasure box and sword.

Personal Comments—16-Year-Old Male with Obsessive Compulsive Disorder

I took all three objects at the mouth of my cave into the interior. The sword was made of gemstone, like lapis lazuli. I went in expecting to see a bat or something of the sort. I expected nothing like the dragon, so much so when I saw it I jumped. I opened the pouch and threw something heavy out of it to turn the dragon's gaze away from me and then I struck it with the sword, not killing it but wounding it slightly. It turned and saw me, I extended the sword from my arm like a warning and defense, he looked me in the face then moved aside allowing me to enter the cavern at the back of the cave. His expression let me know he knew the treasure was for me and that I could have it, and that he was not a foe, and he looked on me with the eyes of a friend. When I entered the back cavern, the treasure room was full of golden coins, ancient weapons, gems and dinosaur skeletons. These dinosaurs were all carnivores and not of the likeness of any known today, except for one very large tyrannosaur skeleton, complete and standing behind the rest of the riches. The others lay strewn in front of and beside the treasure, like scarves wrapping a neck. I took one of the skulls of the dinosaurs in front of me, along with a sword that caught fire when held, some gems and a hand full of coins from the cavern when I knew I had to leave. I walked out past the dragon, and exchanged one final glance with it before coming back to the opening of the cave. When I looked into the meadow, I thought of it as a cave or a meadow in a region of Middle-earth, not in the United States. The fact that a dragon and the ancient weapons of unknown civilizations were in the cave skewed my view of reality and made me question where I was. I exited the cave and entered into the sunlit meadow once again, holding my prize from my entry, and my treasures from within.

Therapeutic Transition

Integration of self with what might be the defiant and restrictive part of self (dragon) to the strong and courageous part of self (distracting and wounding dragon) is evident. Facing the challenge of obsessive-compulsive disorder and working in exposure-and-response cognitive behavioral therapy, this client is learning how to face trials head on and overcome them. Since the dragon is wounded but sees the victor and recognizes the treasure belongs to him and still allows passage is a hopeful sign of strength to overcome and succeed. Exploration of the metaphorical significance of the items taken and discovered could provide discrimination of strengths within self on which to rely during struggles. The uncertainty of the location is normal, as the treatment forces the client to face and eventually overcome the uncertainties associated with OCD. Archetypes and battle drawing would be a strong initiative to follow, perhaps focusing on the armor of strengths that could be worn for the battle.

Creativity Activation

Creativity is first initiated when visualization begins in the imagination during guided imagery as spoken by the therapist. This is further realized when the images are translated from the mind to the page. The medium will also impact the creativity as the individual resonates with its property.

Adaptations for All Guided Imagery

Adaptations relate to the focus in the journey and what is extracted as the symbols for representation. For example, you could add that an object was found in the dwelling, which would allow a variation to the drawings, as the client could represent the new object. The client could also draw an image of self as victorious after the cave exploration. This metaphorical success and image of self could provide further processing for skills and courage to face other challenges. The scripts could be altered slightly for a particular client but should be carefully considered.

Initiative Seventeen—Environmental Awareness

ETC—Cognitive/Symbolic (C/S)
MDV—High Complexity Unstructured Resistive (HCUR)

Therapists have long realized that pathological behaviors are often simply attempts to avoid difficult thoughts and emotions. Unresolved and unrecognized grief, attachment disorders, trauma, and preverbal painful experiences all affect the developing brain. A neurosynaptic pattern is developed very early, perhaps even in the womb, which leads to startle responses, excessive crying or "colic," hypervigilance, lack of reinforcement value, and numerous other "conditions."

We seek to avoid difficult emotions such as unhappiness, fear, or anger. As a result, we do not learn how to use these emotions functionally and to ride through them until they naturally resolve themselves. We therefore learn that certain emotions are not "good" and we should not be experiencing them! People find many ways to avoid uncomfortable emotions—from self-medicating to dissociation.

Mindful awareness, according to Dan Siegel (2012), is a form of awareness in which we are alert and attentive to the present experience without imposing judgments or expectations on it. Mindfulness is a basic human quality, a way of learning to pay attention to whatever is happening in your life that allows you a greater sense of connection to your life inwardly and outwardly. Mindfulness is also a practice, a systematic method aimed at cultivating clarity, insight, and understanding. In the context of your health, mindfulness is a way for you to experientially learn to take better care of yourself by exploring and understanding the interplay of mind and body and mobilizing your own inner resources for coping, growing, and healing (Kabat-Zinn, 2013).

This initiative allows the participant to be aware not only of his or her own body but also of the environment in which it finds itself. The focus on a small component of the external world then is turned back inward to creatively develop a relationship through a fantasy story about that small piece of the world.

Materials

Found objects, poster board, bond paper, colored paper (tissue and construction), glue, paints and variety of brush sizes, oil pastels, pencils, and other mixed media you have available

Directives

1. Weather permitting, go outside and walk slowly, observing what is around you.
2. When something catches your eye, stop and take some time looking at the object. If you can pick it up, take it with you back inside.
3. Create a story about the object. Give your mind free will to be as creative as you can.
4. Write the story.
5. Illustrate the story with the object as central to the composition, using the mixed media of your choice.

Rationale

We are often surprised at the fantasies we are able to create when we do not censor ourselves. This personal fantasy has many symbols, thoughts, and feelings in it. With the therapist or, if in a group, a group member, relate your fantasy as a metaphor of your life right now. There may be glimpses of the past you wish to explore, and that is fine. What materials did you choose to illustrate your fantasy? Why? Be mindful of your body after you have done this initiative. Explore any areas that are uncomfortable, then relax into a breathing stance and put a positive light on the discomfort. What happened?

Figure 6.13 is a pastel drawing of hands, cupped together, holding a stone. There is a background of blue. To the right of the drawing is the

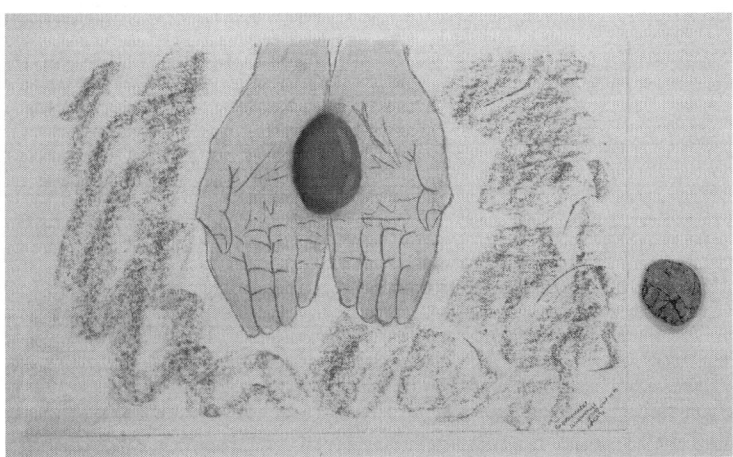

Figure 6.13 Environmental Awareness

stone the young woman found on her walk. She added black lines with a marker to the stone to emphasize cracks that were her own addition.

Personal Comments—20-Year-Old Female Undergraduate Student of Professor Kagin

I was walking around trying to find an object for the environmental awareness project, and I walked past a long landscaped area filled with stones. They all just looked incredibly average, but one stood out because it looked completely smooth. Out of the thousands of stones it was different—and I felt like I could relate to this tiny stone in a weird way, because underneath the smoothness you could see ridges and scratches. I saw that it was once rough and coarse, and it had been roughed-up, but eventually water had washed over it and made it smooth and soft, and I felt like I had been through a similar process in my life, though the roughed-up-ness was life and the raw aspects of my personality, but growing from my experiences and my faith was the water that made it smooth. The creation of the drawing was extremely therapeutic for me, because I felt like I successfully represented how I saw and thought of the stone, and the entire exercise was enjoyable because it was nice to be able to take something so simple from nature and imagine a complex, relatable story for it. It helped me see that everything in the world has a story, and everything is complex and interwoven, even the smallest stone.

Therapeutic Transition

This student was able to see and create the metaphor for her life through the use of an everyday object found outside without any coaxing from a therapist. This experience was cathartic unto itself. The image shows the actual stone that the student used for the story, which she added black lines onto to emphasize the cracks. The student later noted, "I don't know what made me do that, I just did it and it seemed right." This simple statement regarding this action accentuates further the cracks and roughness. Following this story further might allow more insight into *how* the student had developed and/or applied her strength of resiliency. This could be done through drawing, writing, or both.

Creativity Activation

Changing the setting and exploring outside activates the client's senses. Seeking an object begins the process of problem solving. The creativity level is achieved when the found object becomes personified or transformed into a story and the illustration is developed.

Adaptation

Increase the number of images, and give each image a voice (Gestalt). Stay inside or go into a different room to find the object that they have not paid attention to before. For people who lack energy and are feeling depressed, one object could be chosen by the therapist, and each person in the group could write a story and illustrate to show how unique each individual is.

Initiative Eighteen—Box Self (Inner/Outer Self)

ETC—Cognitive/Symbolic (C/S)
MDV—High Complexity Unstructured Restrictive (HCUR)

The use of a prestructured object, the box, to represent the self makes the exercise very concrete. There is an inside and an outside to the box, and translating that to the inner and outer self gives ease to implementation.

Materials

Cardboard box with lid or closure of any size the client chooses. You may wish to assign bringing the box to the session or class or provide the boxes yourself, construction paper, colored tissue paper, magazines, glue, scissors, yarn or twine, feathers, beads, and other miscellaneous décor.

Directives

1. This box is you, your inside self that you may keep hidden and your outside self that others see.
2. Using the materials supplied, create your inner/outer self.
3. Share what you did and any resulting insights. If in a group or even if in a solo session, you may reserve the right to not share certain aspects of your creation. However, note that when you show it, each part will be seen. If a question arises, simply say you are not ready to share this yet.

Rationale

Confronting awareness of different personas we use, this initiative readily involves the client with introspection and symbolic representation of self. The differences between the outside and the inside should give the individual insight into how transparent or repressed he or she is. There is also a protection in this, as the box has a lid and disclosure is a choice.

Figures 6.14 and 6.15 show images of a Box Self project. Figure 6.14 is the outside of the box, with a pink flower on it. Figure 6.15 is the opened box with diagonal lines on the bottom interior and curvilinear lines on the flap of the box.

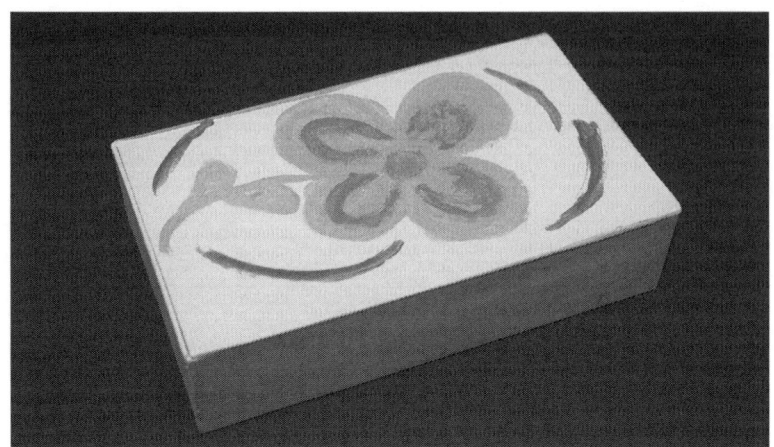

Figure 6.14 Box Self (Inner/Outer Self)

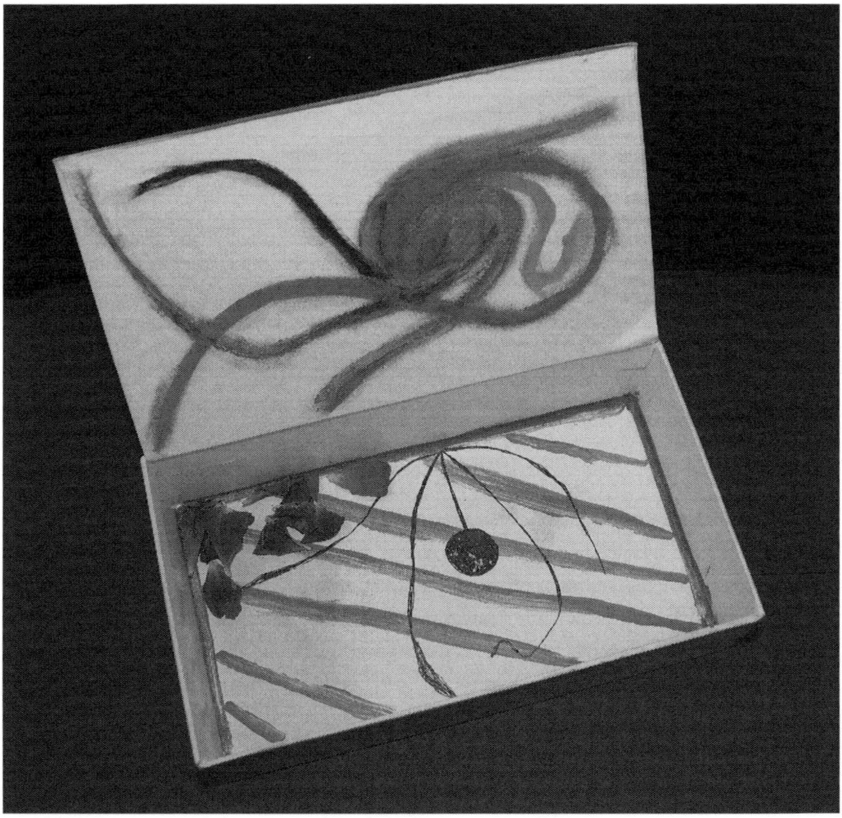

Figure 6.15 Box Self (Inner/Outer Self)

Personal Comments—23-Year-Old Female
Undergraduate Student of Professor Kagin

This is a good exercise for examining self-perception. I became aware of how I think others see me. My inside self represents me outside my prison cell. I am free, dancing, and raw. I have flower petals inside my box because I self-identify with flowers. The purple outline inside my box brings me a feeling of safety. Inside the box I am free to be dancing, raw, and to have self. The knot is what I put between the inside and outside of my box. It is my protection. It is complicated, and colorful. It is how I feel between my inside and outside self. The outside is what others see. This flower is consistent, it is nice. It is plain. It is lifeless. (She reported more in processing that people see her as happy and joyful and outgoing, which was indicated by the large flower on the top of the box. She simply said "this is the inside" but did not elaborate.)

Therapeutic Transition

We believe it would be important for this young lady to be able to feel more comfortable about how she feels and expresses her emotions. Since she works very quickly, one of the directives would be to slow down and elaborate. Ask her to take the images on the inside of the box and paint them on a large piece of paper. If appropriate, ask her to give the box a voice (Gestalt). It would be of particular significance for her to explore the "knot" and even become that twisted intertwined part of herself. There is also something about the outside world that feels unsafe to her. Ask her to add what would make her feel safe and why.

Creativity Activation

The creativity level is achieved when people make choices about materials to be used and how to apply them to the box. The exploration of inside and outside, both physically and mentally, activates creative thinking, as some have color, fabric, or line that move in and out of the box. These decisions are creative solutions.

Adaptation

Possible adaptations include completing the inside self in one session and the outside self in another session to allow for deeper thought and reflection in the creative process. The decision about the boxes is a choice the therapist makes with the client or group and thus impacts the process and brings out different responses. Asking the client to bring in a box versus providing a variety or everyone receiving the same box changes the dynamic. The choice of the box becomes a metaphor for self-image and ego development.

Initiative Nineteen—Body Tracing

ETC—Cognitive/Symbolic (C/S)
MDV—Low Complexity Unstructured Fluid (LCUF)

This is basically a group project and should not be done with just therapist and client alone, as body touching is inevitable. It may also be wise to know whether any of the students or clients have a background in physical or sexual abuse or if anorexia has ever been present. If you are working with a family, note carefully who chooses to trace each person and how it is approached.

Materials

Large sheets of white butcher paper, cut to the length of the person being drawn. Cut two pieces of paper for each person. Provide scissors, watercolor markers, and pastels.

Directives

1. Place the paper on the floor and lie down on it. Choose a stance that depicts your "real" self. Ask a partner to trace your body.
2. On the second piece of paper, ask your partner to trace the position you assume as your "ideal" self.
3. Use the watercolor markers to embellish the figure in whatever manner seems appropriate for "real" and "ideal." This need not be representational, and you may use line, form, and color to depict the two images.
4. When completed, tape the papers to the wall.
5. Going around in a circle, each person stands in front of each drawing and speaks for the drawing using "I am . . ."
6. Process through group feedback.

Rationale

This initiative helps explore how inner feelings translate to body position and body image. It is designed to develop more self-awareness and self-image. The perceived difference between the two may be used strategically to plan for the transition between real and ideal or to help realize that there is no actual difference. The group feedback gives good reflections.

Figure 6.16 shows the image of ideal self drawn by a 22-year-old female. The figure has her hands in her pockets, no face, and one foot on pointed toes.

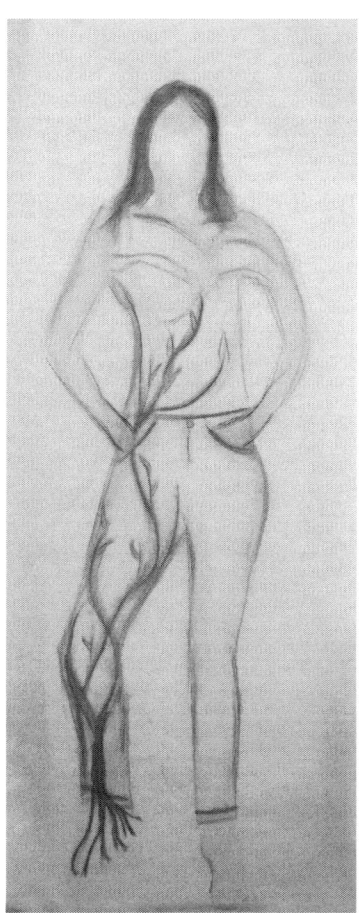

Figure 6.16 Body Tracing

Personal Comments — 22-Year-Old Female Undergraduate Student

I chose pastels because they are the easiest for me to use. I can be free, yet controlled. I love touching the support and blending. I intentionally chose colors for the head as a way of portraying my desire for clarity of mind. I gave myself defined arms because physical strength is important to me. I chose warm, passionate colors to come from my heart/soul reaching out. In general, I gave myself warmth. The pants are jeans which I feel most comfortable and also confident in. However, I made them bolder fun colors because I want to be more daring with how I dress. I drew the vine growing up my leg with roots as my right foot, because being rooted, grounded helps me grow. Then, the way my left foot was positioned when traced lent itself perfectly to be a ballet slipper, which elevated my form like how dance lifts me. On the wall it looks peaceful and comfortable. I seem slightly unfinished. A group member mentioned that my lines are present, my browns too and that I seemed close to my goal. It felt whole to her. I was left with a hard question from my professor about what the face means to me. "Is the omission of the face, because I see it as a mask or because it is too telling?" I have not yet found the answer.

Therapeutic Transition

This student only did the ideal self. Although much of what she said reflects her perception of her real self, it would be a good idea to follow up with the drawing of the real self. She was also left with a question about her identity, as she had not drawn a face. Was this a mask or fear of vulnerability? The new directive to create the real self should include instructions to add the real face.

Creativity Activation

The creativity level is achieved in this initiative when the person is faced with the empty body and is asked to implement symbolism into the ideal self.

Adaptation

Making use of a body template for individual therapy or even for those who are experiencing body image issues would be a safe option, as tracing requires that another person be present.

Initiative Twenty—Lifeline

ETC—Cognitive/Symbolic (C/S)
MDV—High Complexity Structured Resistive (HCSR)

In her book *Expressions of Healing; Embracing the Process of Grief*, Sandra Graves (1994) remarks that most of what we see in our sessions and with our clients stems from unresolved grief and loss. The reason for this is that with every major change in a person's life, there is a loss, and with every loss there is grief. Grief is physical, emotional, intellectual, social, and spiritual. It begins and ends with a neurobiological invasion of hormones that affects each area of life.

Materials

Paper (large, 12 × 18), pencil, colored pencils, markers

Directives

1. Begin by making a "key" in which you designate emotions by color, for example, anger may be red, scared green, happy yellow, or whatever best fits you. This key is placed on a regular piece of bond paper and put aside for later use.
2. The length of the lifeline will depend upon your age and circumstances. It can be changed and added to along the way.
3. Begin with the year of your birth. You will proceed from year to year, writing down what you know or remember or were told about that year. We are especially interested in any major changes each year or events that stand out to you.
4. Your line does not have to be straight or horizontal or vertical but a combination of configurations that best represent that year in your life.
5. After you have written down the main events of that year, go back and select the colors of mad, sad, glad, or scared and apply them as lines or forms in whatever way you wish. You may have all the colors or only one. If you have no memory or "family legend" about that time, then leave the colors off. We have found that the longer this initiative is worked on, the more memories and feelings emerge.
6. Assign an archetype to each period of your life and identify them on the lifeline. Introduce or review the most common archetypes before proceeding with this initiative. You may wish to wait and reflect or do more study on archetypes before completing.

Rationale

This initiative gives a perspective that allows for a great deal of reflective distance. Each year is assessed equally such that whatever traumas or major losses have occurred, they are *part*, not *all* of the lifeline, thus only part of your identity. There have been clients who worked for months on this initiative, so go at their pace. As a pattern of color emerges over the years, be sure to stand back from the work so the colors stand out.

Figures 6.17 and 6.18 show a lifeline with color symbols and written archetypes to support roles and events in life.

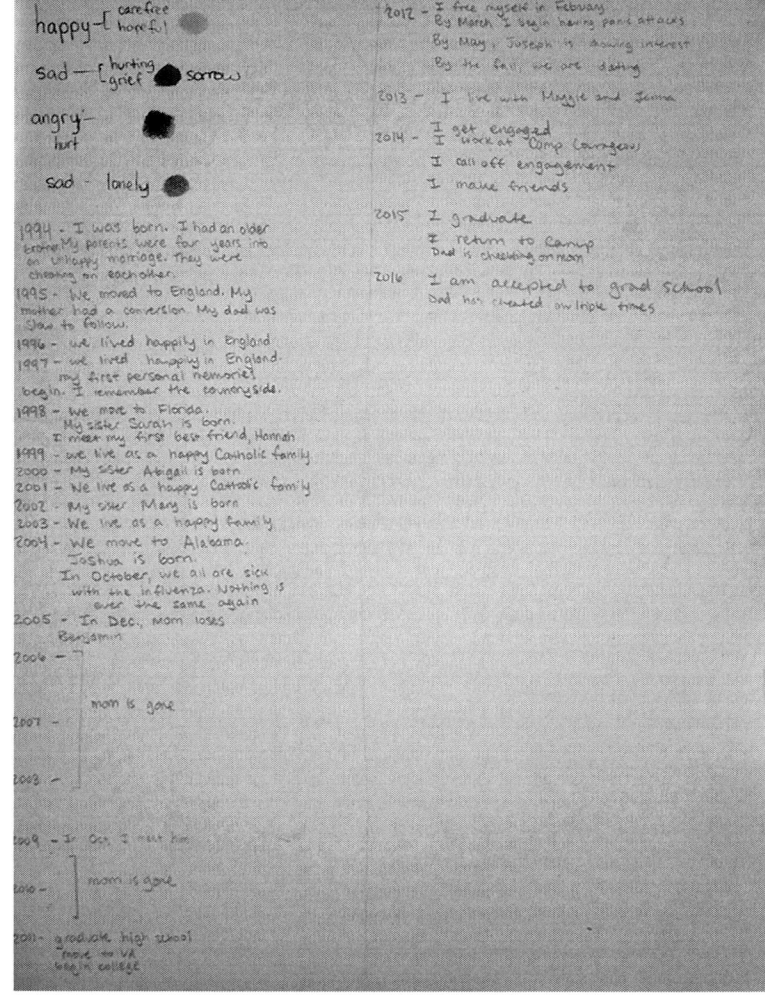

Figure 6.17 Lifeline

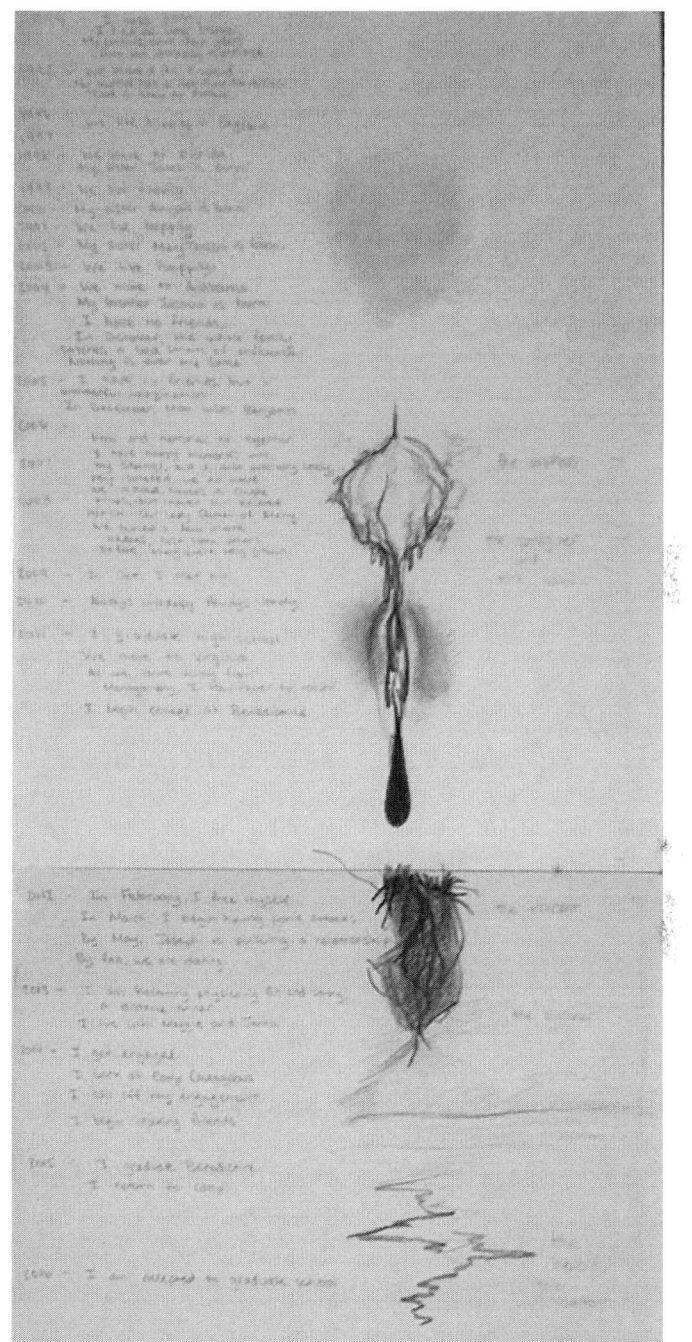

Figure 6.18 Lifeline

Personal Comments—23-Year-Old Female Former Student of Professor Kagin

Here she explores the orphan, the caregiver, and the rebel. Toward the end, she found the innocent, the explorer, and the hero/creator.

I realized that I don't organize my life by years, but by periods marked by events. It wasn't difficult for me to see the "big picture" of my life because of how many times I've played through the major events of my life.

It was strange to see everything together on one timeline. It doesn't even feel like everything has happened in the same life. It feels more like I've been a different person every time. In a way, that's true.

I had much more to write about my early life (that I have little actual memory of) and ended up writing less as I went on. I was surprised by how much I instinctively left out of my more recent years. I could have gone back and added more, especially to 2011–2016, but I left it the way it was.

I was surprised to find I left out a history of positive friendships and relationships. If I were to fill out the timeline more, I would add the names of all the people who I have loved and trusted and have helped me become who I am today.

I didn't think too hard about the images I produced. They were instinctive and impulsive. I'm not satisfied with them, but it's hard to say if that's because they're "wrong" or if it's because they represent a story that's uncomfortable for me to look at.

The archetypes were harder for me to do. I could spend hours analyzing, but I went with my immediate gut reaction. I identified archetypes with periods of life rather than years, so that's how I wrote them.

I wrote with a pencil. I don't usually write with pencil, but I felt the need to leave the option to erase things. In the end, I made no major changes to content.

Therapeutic Transition

The addition of the archetypes in the timeline, marking the time period, was a positive follow-up to this initiative. The young woman was able to identify the roles at times in her life. A good next step would be to explore these roles in significance to her role today: creator. This could be done through drawings of each and an examination of their attributes. What has the creator kept? What are the strengths from the trials? The creation of persona masks would allow exploration of these archetypes and role-playing or even Gestalt processing for deeper awareness.

Creativity Activation

Linear thinking often leans one toward the cognitive, so telling the client to create any format with a beginning and end that corresponds with the feelings associated with that period of life awakens new awareness and creative responses.

Adaptation

You may wish to precede this initiative for number Twenty-One. Have the client choose a particularly emotional time of life from their lifeline and write an autobiographical description of that experience. Also, creating a graph of the emotional key would be very enlightening. Movement or sound could also be translated from a particular area of the timeline, or one could orchestrate the entire lifeline. Videotape the performance and process with the client.

Initiative Twenty-One—12 Archetypes and My Roles in Life

ETC—Cognitive/Symbolic (C/S)
MDV—High Complexity Structured Resistive (HCSR)

This initiative explores Jungian archetypes and how they are used by each of us during our lifespan. The beginning of this section outlines the 12 archetypes that are discussed extensively by Carl Jung in numerous publications, which are preparatory information for the completion of the initiative My Roles in Life.

It was Jung's belief that there is a collective unconscious, from which we all inherit particular patterns of behavior or traits. These archetypes may be seen in ancient and contemporary myths common to the human race, not just within a given culture, and they give a structure for each of us to explore and to ascertain which are most fitting. The patterns or types within the archetypes also help us understand ourselves better and learn to cope with our own particular personalities.

Jung originally looked at the basic framework of the archetypes (a concept he borrowed from Plato): *anima, animus*, self, and other (the shadow). Each of the 12 most common archetypes relates to a function, an emotion, a problem, a response to a task, a gift, and a virtue (Jung, 1968). The shadow side of each archetype must also be considered (Pearson, 1991, 1998). Remind your client, yourself, and your students that there is no "up" without a "down" and that all symbols and archetypes are bivalent. If handled correctly, exploring the opposites and emphasizing the positive have great and lasting results.

An in-depth study of the archetypes is advised. You will not find it in this book; rather, we have summarized in lay language the roles these personas have in our lives. A person may have been born with a specific propensity for one or two of the archetypes, but life has its way of calling for resilience and developing new insights and skills.

Jung divided the archetypes into three developmental categories: the Ego types (Innocent, Orphan, Hero, and Caregiver), the Soul types (Explorer, Rebel, Lover, and Creator), and the Self types (Jester, Sage, Magician, Ruler; Jung, 1968).

The Archetypes

The Innocent: A desire to get to paradise and be happy defines this archetype. There is a feeling of freedom to be whoever you are. The

Innocent has a strategy to do things right but a weakness to be boringly innocent. The strength of this ego type is its faith and optimism.

The Orphan: Has a need to belong and is thought of as the regular guy or gal. The Orphan connects with others, and his greatest fear is to be left out. The Orphan is down to earth, solid as a rock. A strength of being realistic, empathetic, and genuine is compelling.

The Hero: As part of our transformation from childhood to adulthood, the Hero emerges as a desire to prove one's worth through courageous, sometimes dangerous acts. The acting-out adolescent is a shadow character of this warrior. The Hero's goal is to master in a way that improves the world, and his greatest fear is weakness and vulnerability. The Hero's strategy is to be as strong and competent as possible.

The Caregiver: This persona wants to help others, sometimes to a fault. The greatest fear of the Caregiver is to be selfish or lack gratitude. Martyrdom is often a result of overdoing this role in life, and it is easy for the caregiver to become the victim. Its greatest strength is compassion and generosity.

The Explorer (Seeker): A desire to discover oneself through exploring the world has the goal of a more fulfilling life. Being trapped or feeling inner emptiness is the greatest fear of the Seeker. The shadow side of the explorer is the misfit who wanders aimlessly (the Gypsy of the soul). The strategy of the Explorer is to seek out and experience new things. The Explorer's strength is autonomy, ambition, and being true to one's soul.

The Rebel (Destroyer): The Rebel seeks revolution or revenge and has a desire to make right what is not working. Powerlessness is the Rebel's greatest fear, which can lead to compensatory shadow, destruction, or turning to crime. The Rebel leads in the strategy to disrupt, destroy, or shock. The Rebel's strength lies in being outrageous through radical freedom fighting.

The Lover: Seeking intimacy and experience, the Lover's goal is being in relationship with the people and surroundings they love. Being alone or unwanted is the greatest fear, which can lead the Lover to please others at the risk of his own identity. The Lover is passionate and forgiving, but too much striving toward these goals can lead to obsession and compulsion.

The Creator: A strong desire to create things of lasting value leads the Creator toward realizing a vision. The Creator develops artistic creativity and imagination. Its weakness is perfectionism and bad solutions with a fear of having the vision be only mediocre at best.

The Jester (Trickster): Having a great time, lighting up the world, being the life of the party are characteristics of the Jester. He lives in the moment and is playful, joking, and funny. His greatest fear is to be boring. The Jester's weakness is frivolity and wasting time. His shadow is sneaking and stealth-like.

The Sage: A truth seeker, the Sage or wise man or woman uses intelligence and analysis to understand the world and the meaning of life. The Sage seeks truth through self-reflection and thinking. The Sage is wise but must be careful about too much study and no action. Its greatest fear is being misled or ignorant.

The Magician: A goal of making dreams come true and understanding the fundamental laws of the universe lead the Magician to develop a vision and live by it. The shadow side of this persona is the manipulator, but the strength of this archetype is the ability to find solutions that suit all. This archetype has been also known as the Healer, Medicine Man, or Shaman.

The Ruler: The Ruler desires and strives for control. Prosperity and success are its goal. The ability to exercise power is its strategy and leadership its talent. The other side of this persona is the malevolent dictator. The weakness of the Ruler is the inability to delegate, thus taking on too much to handle and failing in its striving.

My Roles in Life

Directives

1. Review your Lifeline initiative.
2. Decide which archetype fits best with various roles in your life as a child, teen, adult (wife, mother, student, professional, or others).
3. Develop a chart dividing significant events and years.
4. Below the year, write the archetypal role you have played in a significant event(s) of that year.

See Figure 6.19 for example by former graduate student of Dr. Graves-Alcorn.

Rationale

Archetypes are very useful in giving guidance to clients and students. Since it is also a universal language, it ties cultures and periods of time together; thus we are not just isolated beings. The archetypes' roles also change throughout lifetime development, and a shadow "self" can be recognized so that the positive hero can emerge.

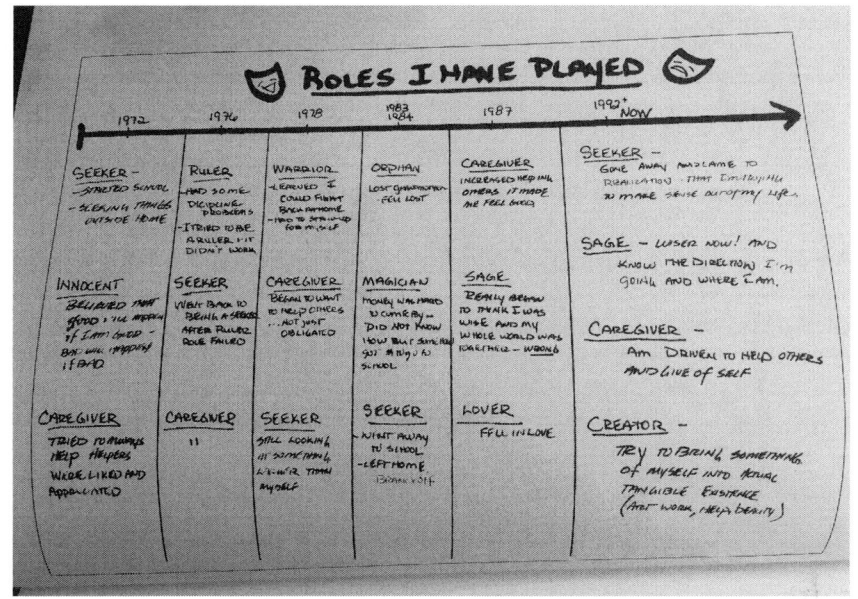

Figure 6.19 My Roles in Life and the 12 Archetypes

Therapeutic Transition

The next step in exploring the archetypes would be to become one or two of the personas identified. Persona masks (Initiative Twenty-Two) is an excellent follow-up.

Creativity Activation

This initiative is very thought provoking, and the creativity occurs when the generalized archetype is personalized and placed in a given time and circumstance.

Adaptation

Choose a challenge and pick a partner who reminds you of the persona attached to that challenge. Role-play the scene of the challenge.

Initiative Twenty-Two—Persona Masks—Anima and Animus: the Shadow Self

ETC—Cognitive/Symbolic (C/S)
MDV—High Complexity Unstructured Fluid or Resistive (HCUF or R), a mid-range of fluid

According to Jung (1968), the anima and animus lead us to our shadow selves and help us to understand both our feminine and masculine components from early development through the lifespan. The shadow self can be sadistic and cruel or compassionate and loving. Each persona we embody is given a choice as to which "side" will be expressed. If we also investigate these ego states with a known archetype, we are able to ascertain each role we have chosen and delve into its inception, perhaps to make a different choice.

Materials

Mixed-media items—any available: glue, scissors, variety of colors and textures of paper, markers, paint, yarn, beads, buttons, found objects, fabric, wire, etc.

Directives

1. Create two masks that represent conflicting sides of self.
2. Process, considering the integration of self and the importance of each side.

Rationale

This initiative challenges the client to identify and acknowledge two conflicting sides of self and examine the differences between them. The creation of a mask as the means to represent self allows for the personification of the characteristic. This promotes the understanding of the differing sides of self, how a client might use or hide parts of self, and how to integrate or recognize areas that need to be addressed. Day-to-day feelings, responses, and behaviors can be identified. Examination of each side of self facilitates integration of the self and understanding of the importance of having each role and how it helps and/or hinders. Recognizing the conflicting sides rather than just two parts of self forces the client to engage with challenging elements of self, so necessary in developing insight.

Figures 6.20 and 6.21 show the two sides of one mask created by a woman challenged by integration of her feminine and masculine selves. Figure 6.20 is the masculine side, with red and black signifying anger. Figure 6.21 is the feminine side, which is more nurturing and serene in purple and blue.

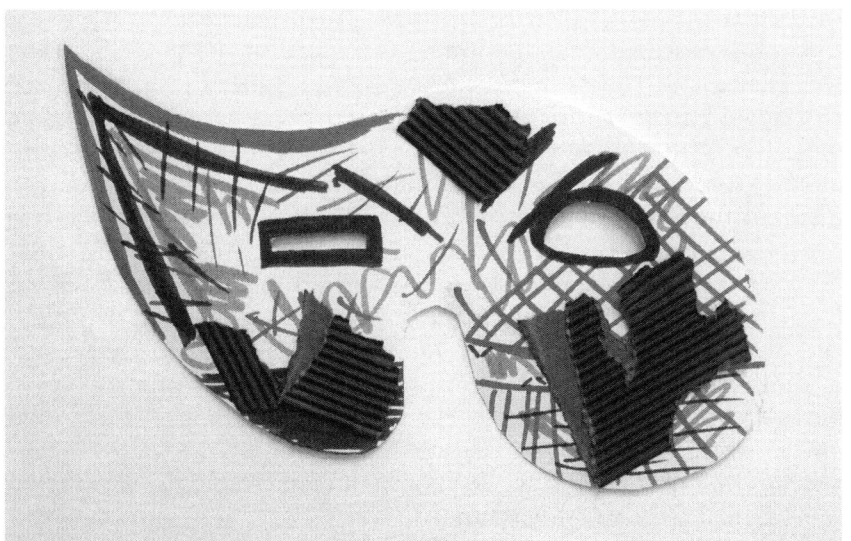

Figure 6.20 Persona Masks

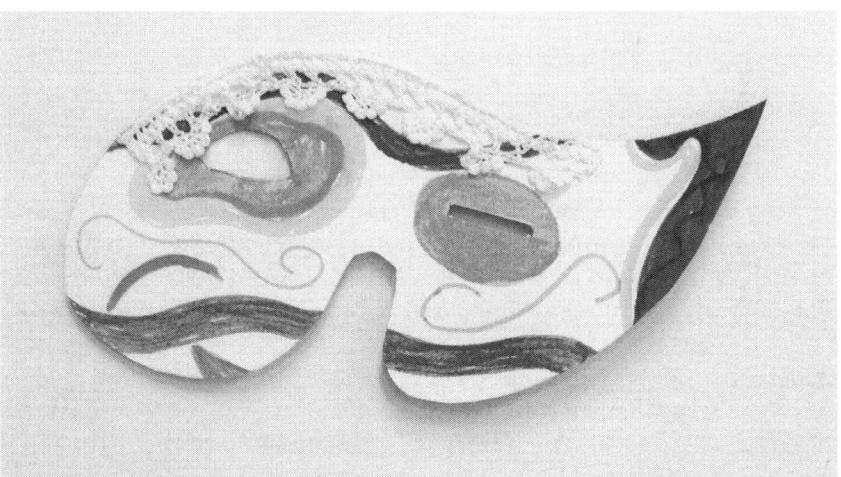

Figure 6.21 Persona Masks

Personal Comments—21-Year-Old Female
Student of Professor Kagin
This was a fun project even though it dealt with an inner conflict. Since I decided to do two sides of the same mask, it helped me to see the unity and blending of the two sides of my self—my mother's and father's influences that make me who I am. It was reaffirming that I was able to make them fit together so well. It helped me to objectively look at the sides and see them for what they are.

During processing, discussion of the shape of the masks and the soft curves and sharp angles were explored. One side of the mask represented anger, strong drive, and judgment (the negative anima), the other nurturing and gentleness (the positive animus). She commented that when she decided to make one mask instead of two and then cut the desired shape of her mask from Bristol paper, she was concerned about how the two would be able to work with the variations. However, as she processed, she realized that the sharp angle on the masculine side was dominated by the harsh angle and helped to emphasize the edge of the anger, but the curve allowed the softer side of that to be evident. Likewise, on the feminine side, the soft curve made up the significant parts of the mask, and the angle, which lifted upward, could be seen as uplifting. Both sides have a textural component, intentionally placed to represent elements of the conflicting sides. One is rigid with lines and torn edges like anger; one is lace, soft and delicate like the gentleness discussed. She felt that the way each side was able to make use of elements of the other helped to unify the mask (and herself), and she felt good about this discovery.

Therapeutic Transitions

This young woman addressed an angry and determined side of self, recognizing the challenges of that part and where it had come from (father), as well as the feminine and passive side of self that could perhaps be too eager to help and serve others to a fault. Acknowledging these qualities within herself and where they had come from but also integrating them into a single mask (back and front) was useful. While dialoging with the masks is often a step used in processing with this initiative, the integration of the two into one limited this use of the masks. Therefore, a further exploration of how these two sides, though able to unify, still have a strong conflict would be useful. This could be done by the creation of a second mask set or of a variation on the battle drawing, where each side is represented in a conflict and the roles are explored. Furthermore, a possible self-portrait with elements of both could be created as she integrates and accepts these parental parts into herself and takes ownership of them. She identified the sharp, pointed edge on the masculine mask as aggressive but the same sharp edge as uplifting on the feminine side. Helping her to find ways to recognize the strengths of these characteristics and how to manage them in appropriate and self-promoting ways would be integrative and empowering.

Creativity Activation

Following the cognitive decisions of which sides of self to create and exploration of those sides, the client begins to make decisions about the roles. With each decision about materials and how the mask will actually "look," creativity increases. The masks are not required to visually represent faces and therefore can be functional masks or nonfunctional. Each executed decision leads to the next, enhancing creativity and encouraging symbolic use of color and materials. The end product can be worn or not, but the creativity that fed the process allows for abstract exploration of parts of self and thereby increases reflection on attributes of self. Creative decision making occurs when clients create a mask of raw materials, shaping, embellishing, and wearing elements that represent parts of self but are not materials actually worn on a face. This symbolic representation of conflicting sides of self requires creative thought and activation to make the intangible tangible.

Adaptations

While this initiative calls for the creation of two masks, as the student quoted mentioned, one way to adapt it is to make one mask with two sides to represent the conflicting sides. This especially facilitates a unification of parts, which might be the goal for a client in recognizing strengths and weaknesses that are in conflict.

Additionally, the use of a prefabricated mask that could be decorated would be useful so the client could physically put on the mask and it would conform to the shape of the face. This has also been done with masks that are made of plaster gauze from the client's face directly, and one or two could be made. If made this way, the inside could be an inside conflict, whereas the outside could be a part of self that needs to be expressed. This distance might be helpful for psychodrama use in sessions. If the personification of self is volatile for a client, hats could be substituted.

Initiative Twenty-Three—Battle Drawing

ETC—Cognitive/Symbolic (C/S)
MDV—Low Complexity Unstructured Fluid (LCUF) or Resistive (R)

The battle represents inner conflicts with which the individual deals, often on a daily basis. This initiative asks the participant to identify and focus on just one of those conflicts.

Materials

Paint (watercolor or tempera), brushes of many sizes, water, paper towels, drawing paper, cray-pas (oil pastels) or markers

Directives

1. Think of your greatest conflict in life at this moment.
2. Decide which archetypes are involved in the conflict.
3. Draw a battle between two archetypes, one the antagonist and the other the protagonist, representing them in whatever images you choose to create. It is possible to identify more than one archetype for the protagonist and antagonist.

Rationale

This initiative should be done after previous exploration of archetypes has been done. The images will be compared for powerfulness, space used, size, and impact of the battle. Is there actually a battle depicted? Are there any weapons? Do the protagonist and antagonist touch? Who wins? This allows the participant to get reflective distance on a highly emotional issue and put it into symbolic form.

Figure 6.22 is a Battle painting between water and ground painted in representational colors, completed by Author Two, Christa Kagin.

Personal Comments—Author Two, Christa Kagin

When I started this project the only visual I had was a wave and I saw it in a variety of ways and I knew that it was the element I was battling. The question then was what will represent me? I began to write some words related to water and its effects—flooding, erosion, deep, powerful. Then I had to decide what I was. Immediately I wrote the word resilient, and I thought what thing does the water have a relationship with that it also battles. The answer, of course, was land, specifically a mountain, strong and powerful that stands

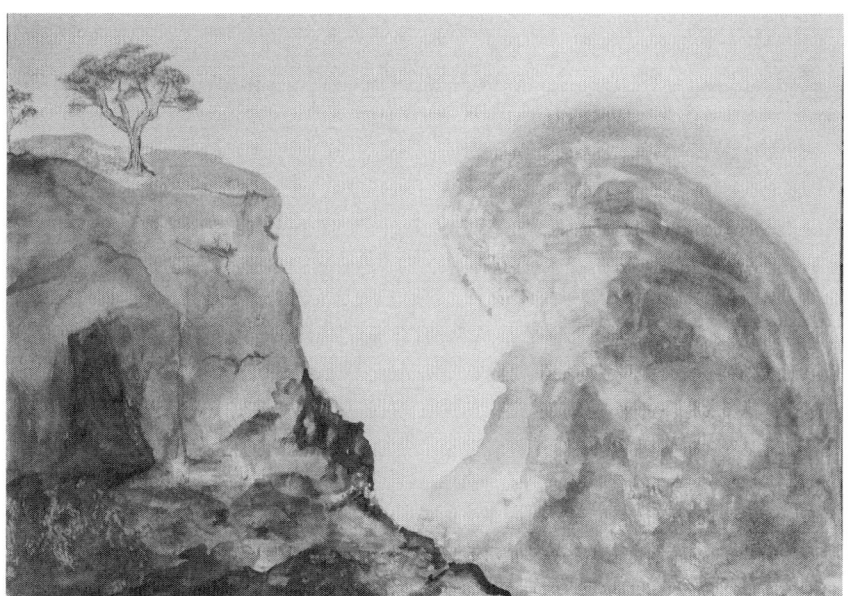

Figure 6.22 Battle Drawing

the test of time. Though the waters wash over it, sometimes eroding and making changes, flooding and washing it out, saturating it, the water also always recedes and the mountain still stands, slightly altered, forever changed, but nonetheless strong. On this land is where life is abundant, rooted deep like the tree and though the storms of the water may come, the tree still stands tall in the sun, weathered by battles but growing ever upward. In my painting the wave is huge, nearly as tall as the height of the tree on the mountain, but not quite, and when the curl moves in and comes down it will never touch the plateau or the tree. I recognize that I have chosen an antagonist that cannot just be slain and left behind. On the contrary I have chosen one that only settles down and then in time will build up momentum and power and rage again. But during that time life will be renewed on the mountain. This is the hope that keeps me going. I see this battle as between the archetypes of the creator and the warrior (water) and the seeker and the sage (mountain).

Therapeutic Transition

Given the insight of this woman, I (Author One, Graves-Alcorn) would ask her to do the persona masks of each of the archetypes she has identified. Then she would speak with the mask on and give that archetype a voice, saying "I am."

Creativity Activation

Creativity occurs first when the decision is made how to represent the antagonist and the protagonist and is fully developed as the battle begins to take shape on the page.

Adaptation

Prior to using this initiative, direct the client to do a drawing of the protagonist preparing for battle and giving it more power.

Initiative Twenty-Four—Powerful and Powerless Collage

ETC—Cognitive/Symbolic (C/S)
MDV—High Complexity Unstructured Resistive (HCUR)

This initiative is multifaceted in use. We all experience a sense of helplessness, thus powerlessness, from time to time throughout our lives. This is true through all stages of life as we transition and grow. We also experience self-empowerment when challenges are overcome, battles are won, or excellence is recognized. It is especially notable when change takes place and adaptation is the result. You will find it intriguing when you process your work, as sometimes the distinction between powerful and powerless is totally lost and they are the same—a bivalence that life always presents to us.

Materials

Poster board or large drawing paper (2 pieces), pictures from magazines, glue, and scissors. Be sure to have a variety of magazines available.

Directives

1. Look through as many magazines as possible or available, choosing a "second glance" at an image that appears either powerful or powerless to you. If you question which it is, cut or tear it out anyway. Gather as many images as possible.
2. On the first poster board, select images for Powerless and place them on the board. When you are satisfied with the arrangement, glue them down.
3. On the second poster board, select images for Powerful and place them on the board. When you are satisfied, glue them down.
4. If time is not a factor, make this a homework assignment, taking as long as needed.

Rationale

As we explore our thoughts and feelings, the use of cognitive problem solving often leads to new insights. The images are concrete yet can be symbolic. In fact, this initiative yields a more symbolic response when meaning is put on a picture you have decided made you feel powerful or powerless.

Figures 6.23 and 6.24 are the images for Powerful and Powerless collages. Powerful (Figure 6.23) is marked by full use of the page, with

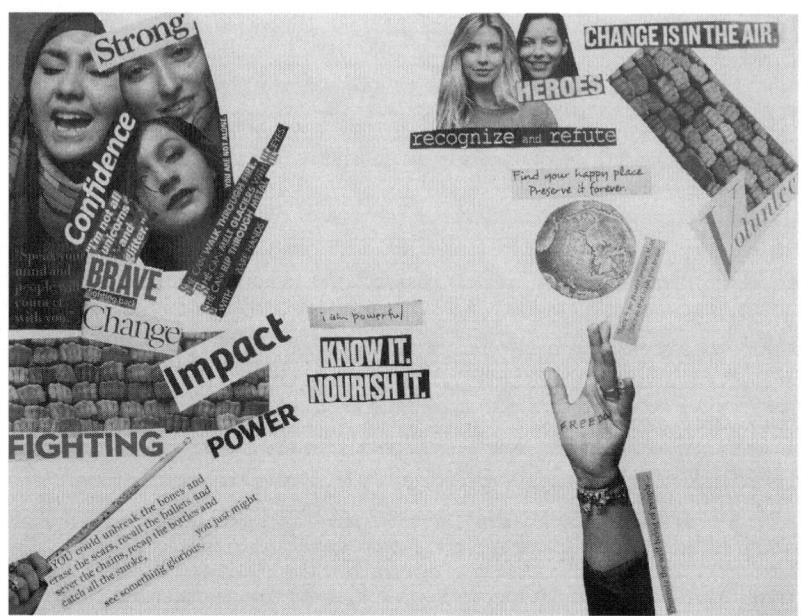

Figure 6.23 Powerful and Powerless Collage (Powerful)

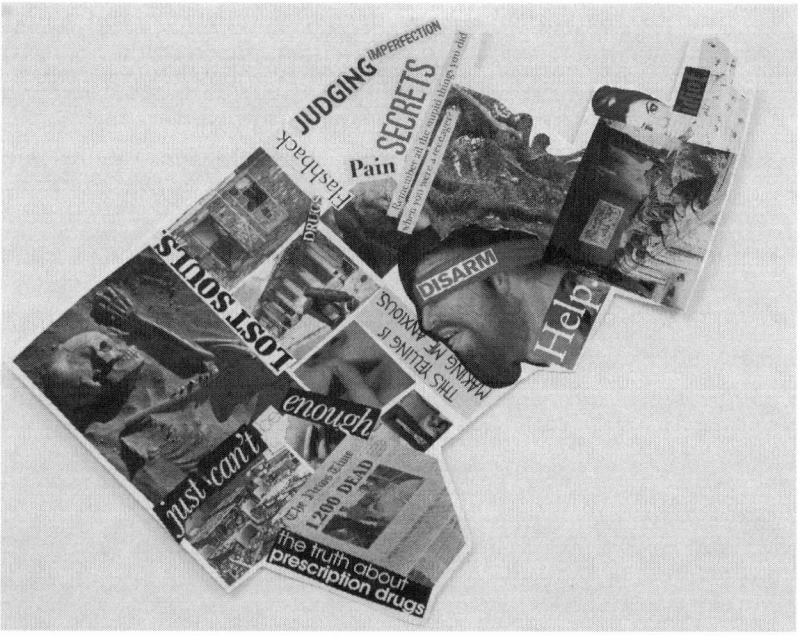

Figure 6.24 Powerful and Powerless Collage (Powerless)

some negative space. Powerless (Figure 6.24) is contained in a strong diagonal overlapping of images down the middle of the page.

Personal Comments—22-Year-Old Female
Student of Professor Kagin

Powerful/Powerless
Creating these collages was one of my favorite directives I have done. While looking through the magazines I noticed it was difficult to find images that were truly powerful. A lot of things were displayed in a way that was trying to make it seem powerful but were images that promoted poor self-esteem. I began being more attracted to words and phrases and how I could rearrange them in a poetic way, a way that showed true strength. I began to get frustrated searching for powerful images and quickly shifted into focusing on powerless. Instead of focusing on powerlessness in general I focused on things that have made me powerless. In my collage my battle with drugs and suicide is evident and is referenced through images and phrases, ironically the phrases were taken from articles glorifying drugs. As I began to feel my collage was finished there was still so much white on the paper so I decided to cut out everything I had collaged and place it in the middle of a new large white piece of paper. This seemed right to me not only because my images were centered but this now showed how being powerless makes me feel small and isolated. Then I returned to my powerful collage; here the struggle began. I searched and searched but I could not find enough images to cover the page and became quite frustrated. I was happy with the words and poetry I had created and the images I had found but it didn't seem to be enough. My powerful collage shows the power of being a woman and the strength of overcoming personal battles. It speaks a strong message when read and looked at closely but the overall visual is incomplete. If I could, I would spend time on this, I would keep working on this collage until I was happy with the entire message.

Therapeutic Transition

Since the visual search for powerful images fell short, it would be good for the client to explore her own idea of powerfulness through drawing or painting. Identifying what was lacking in the magazine images and exploring these attributes in self would be helpful. What was missing? Do you have that in you? How do you (or would you) show that to the world? What can increase powerfulness in self?

Creativity Activation

From the beginning of this set of directives, the exploration of images and how to make them represent something other than what they are representing is a creative act. Thinking about the visual of an archeological dig and translating that into a metaphorical image of powerfulness or powerlessness fosters creativity. Further exploring the relationship of contrasting images to one another activates creative thinking and problem solving. It is this element of visual production that allows any material or image to become a catalyst for creativity and therefore a new way of seeing and thinking.

Adaptations

This initiative could be explored by drawing images of Powerful and Powerless when magazines are not available for the collage aspect. Processing could then include discussion of colors that symbolically represent power and weakness, lines that look powerful or weak, and compositional placement and scale of objects.

Initiative Twenty-Five—Rhyne's Problem-Solving Collage

ETC—Cognitive/Symbolic (C/S) and Perceptual/Affective (P/A)
MDV—High Complexity Structured Resistive (HCSR)

This initiative uses elements of design, which is an aesthetic experience, combined with exploration of symbolism for problem solving, information retrieval, and developing a new perspective.

Materials

Construction paper, 12 × 18 sheet of paper, sheet of notebook or copy paper, pencil, glue stick, scissors

Directives

1. Identify a problem or struggle you are facing right now.
2. Identify specific elements of this problem/issue.
3. Assign the elements different shapes. They can be geometric shapes or abstract shapes.
4. Create a key for the shapes.
5. Cut out the shapes from construction paper.
6. Put the key away.
7. Arrange the shapes into a composition that is aesthetically pleasing without giving thought to the key or the problem. Glue them down.
8. Process the collage by first looking at the way you have placed the shapes together on the page.
9. Process the collage secondly by identifying the elements of the problem with the key. Take note of what elements are placed next to, overlapping, and distant from one another. Give heed to the color used, size of each shape, and placement on the page.
10. How does the arrangement of the pieces help to give you a new insight into the problem? How does the placement, scale, color give you insight into the elements of the problem? Are you surprised by the size of one element because perhaps you saw that as more insignificant to the issue?
11. Analyze the collage with another for objective observations. How does this change your perspective on the problem?

Rationale

Breaking down a problem into specific parts and then again assigning them abstract representation (shapes only) facilitates the exploration of the problem into isolated and manageable elements. The simple act of dissecting the issue can often provide insight. However, with Rhyne's Problem-Solving Collage, the insight is driven further through abstract representation, separation from meaning, and complete visual exploration. The aesthetic placement of the parts of the problem into a single visual collage, separate from thinking about the problem, provides distance and creates a whole from the pieces. Seeing a problem from multiple vantages and configured in a new way helps process, organize, and also see solutions.

Figure 6.25 shows the finished collage of both abstract and representational shapes representing the problem of a challenging friendship that needed resolution.

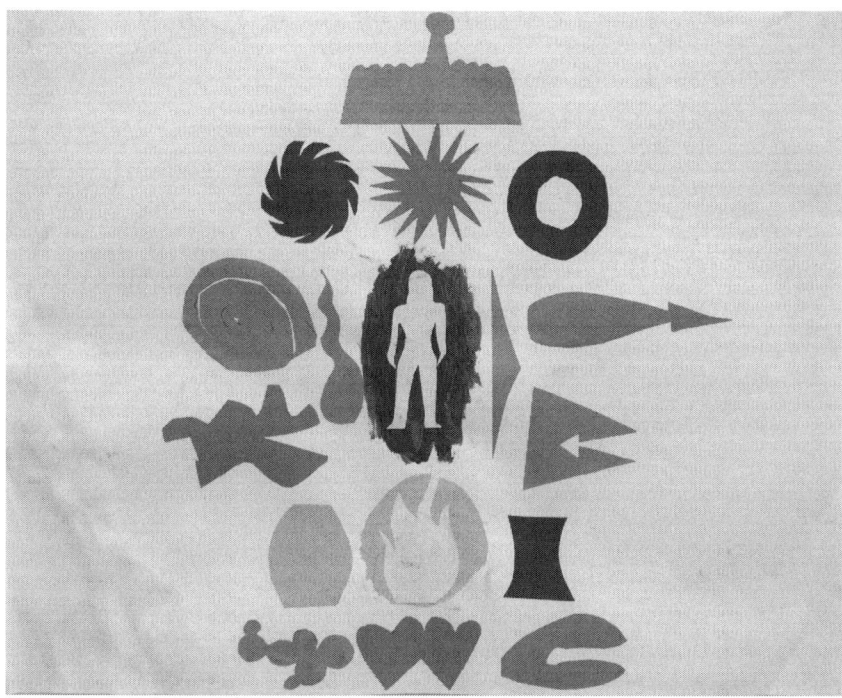

Figure 6.25 Rhyne's Problem-Solving Collage

Personal Comments — 19-Year-Old Female
Student of Professor Kagin

The problem was my friend that was being expelled for bad choices she had made involving the school, and I wasn't sure how to deal with it—whether to try and end the friendship or whether to hold on. In my head, before the exercise, I had unidentifiable emotions, worries, thoughts and questions swirling in my brain too fast for me to keep still, identify the situation and find a solution. This exercise helped me a lot because, with each key, I was able to assign a problem to a shape, freeze it and stop it from swirling around in my brain, put it aside and find the next emotion/question/worry/thought. The shapes in the key didn't have much significance, I only made the first shape that came to mind—I mostly used the shapes just as labels to help me organize the problem. Eventually I had all the different components of the problem assigned to a shape or key, and they were out of my brain and on these shapes instead. Then I was able to organize the problem and assign relevance or importance of the component of the problem in the shapes' proximity to the figure of the woman, who was my friend. Eventually I was able to evaluate and weigh the worth and value of the friendship against the cost it was having on me and my life, and was able to find a solution to my problem much more easily. This exercise helped me find a solution to a very heavy problem in my life, and it helped me way more than I originally thought it was going to. After this exercise I was able to manage the situation much more practically and with a much more level head.

Creativity Activation

Creativity is activated when shapes become the representation of parts of a problem. Their abstraction and simplification of the parts encourages creativity. Furthermore, aesthetically creating a compositional whole with the shapes and thinking about how the shapes work together requires creative thinking, shifting the creativity to a higher level. The problem is reevaluated once the collage is complete and seeing something anew creates a change.

Adaptations

While this initiative is successful in its function as it is, there are a few ways it could be changed that might serve one client better than another. Limiting the color of the construction paper would help a client see that all of the parts belong to a whole. Moreover, adding papers with textures could allow a client to provide a new emphasis on a particular part of the issue, giving variety. Waiting to glue pieces to the page would allow the client to move them around and discuss their relationships and placement to explore the problem from multiple views. A second benefit to not gluing but saving the pieces for a later session would allow a client to process and explore any efforts they've put into addressing the problem and to adjust by changing or subtracting parts in a new aesthetic assembly.

Initiative Twenty-Six—Family-of-Origin Sculpture

ETC—Cognitive/Symbolic (C/S)
MDV—Low Complexity Structured Resistive (LCSR)

This initiative is a tactile experience of creation that facilitates a client's complete immersion in the therapeutic process of examining and feeling the roles of the family on self. Both the way in which the materials are used and the materials themselves and also the way the product is processed promotes a sense of awareness and raw emotive response.

Materials

Plasticine clay in all colors: skin tones, primaries and secondaries, black, white, grays

Directives

1. Ask each participant to create a symbol for each family member and then to combine them into a single family sculpture.
2. Ask client to consider the roles and interactions of each.
3. Once the sculptures have been created, clients will process the family sculpture by asking group members to "play the role" of a particular family member.
4. Each member will then describe the way it *feels* to be in the family sculpture and describe the relationship his/her particular family member symbol has to the others.
5. Group members can move or rearrange the symbols into a new configuration.
6. The client will process his/her responses to the descriptions and changes.

Rationale

This initiative allows participants to look at and explore their family objectively to discover possible dynamics and identify feelings and relationships with family members. Allowing the group members the opportunity to "be" a member of the family, describing and expressing how it feels to be as they are in the sculpture, and providing an opportunity for the rearrangement of members creates the possibility for new insights into the family and one's role in it.

Figure 6.26 is a plasticine clay sculpture of six multicolored balls placed on a light-colored base.

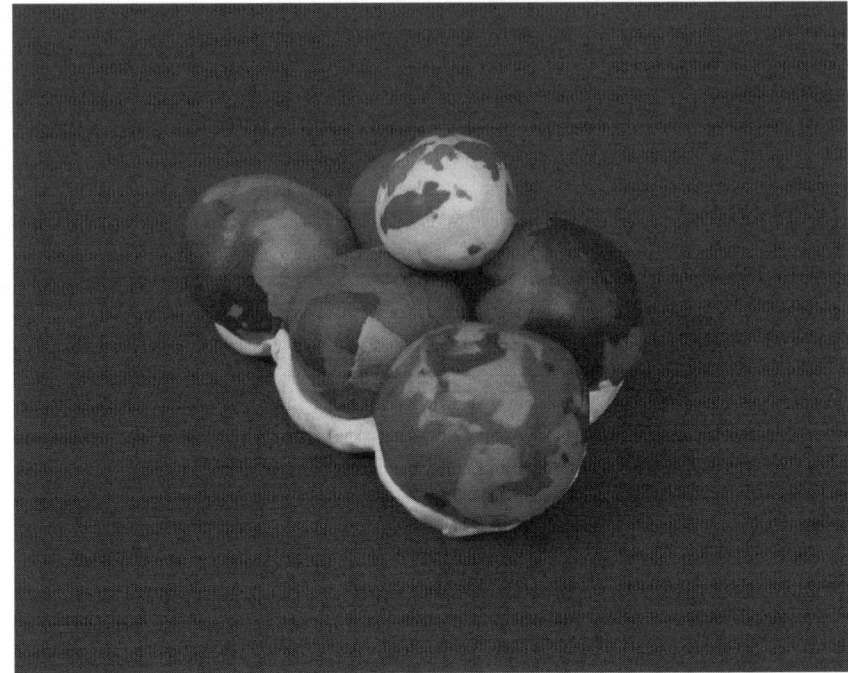

Figure 6.26 Family Sculpture

Personal Comments—21-Year-Old Female
Student of Professor Kagin

It was very useful to have a 3-D representation of my family unit so that I could analyze it better. It was frustrating assigning group members the role of my family members because they don't know them past (beyond) how I've described them. I also couldn't configure my sculpture to accurately show the relationships between all my family members.

Therapeutic Transition

For this young woman, an adaptation and elaboration of the family sculpture might be a good option. Reconfiguring the sculpture and separating each family member then placing the figures on the table in an order that better identifies the relationships to each family member could help to resolve her frustration with the current state of the sculpture. This would also facilitate discussion of variations in relationships and why. How does the new configuration better represent her family?

Creativity Activation

Creativity activation begins when participants begin to create symbols or visual representations for family members. It is furthered when group members are assigned roles and must represent family for the client and also when the members role-play as other members' families. The role-playing element of this initiative helps to foster more creativity and thus can impact the resolution the members experience as they process family roles and integrate understanding of self within the family unit.

Adaptations

It is possible for the client to role-play each family member for the group and then receive feedback from the group on what they hear and notice in body language and projections of personalities. It would be possible to avoid the assignment of roles to group members and still get feedback from them on roles by exploring the sculptures strictly from the perspective of "relationships" they see in the forms represented. Writing changes on paper from this adaptation rather than speaking them might allow for more reflection on the part of the client even beyond the group session.

Initiative Twenty-Seven—Survival on an Island

ETC—Cognitive/Symbolic (C/S)
MDV—High Complexity Structured Resistive (HCSR)

This is one of the most widely used initiatives for workshops and introductory seminars on art therapy or in the classroom, as well as an excellent team-building tool. The manner in which each person attempts to "survive" and develop as part of a new social order is very intriguing and can also be quite confrontational.

Materials

Construction paper, markers, pastels, butcher paper, glue, scissors

Directives

1. Position yourself so that you are comfortable in your chair. Relax your body. Begin to breathe deeply and clear your mind.
2. Today you are going to participate in a guided imagery. Close your eyes and continue to focus on your breathing. Prepare for a journey.
3. Imagine you are on a cruise. You are sailing in Caribbean waters. You can hear the ocean, you can feel the sun, you feel relaxed. You are enjoying yourself. This is a wonderful day. Suddenly you hear a horn blow, and someone says over the sound system that there is a small problem with the ship, but everything should be okay. You return to your blissful experience, not worried at all. After a short time, the horn sounds again and the voice says that the ship will need to be evacuated. Guests should prepare to board the lifeboats. There has been a call for assistance, and everyone will be rescued, but they must evacuate at this time. Look around you. Prepare to leave the ship. Quickly choose three things that you will take with you. Pause. Now board the lifeboat and prepare to leave the ship. There are six to eight people in the boat with you. Be assured that you are not in peril. As the boat lowers into the water, notice the difference in sounds as the water laps against the small vessel. Begin to travel away from the ship. Pause. After a while, you see land before you, so you row harder and prepare to be on dry land again. Finally you reach the sandy beach. You get out of the boat, taking your three items with you. You are safely on land.

4. Using construction paper only, create the three items you took with you off of the ship.
5. (The remainder of this can be completed in another session.)
6. With a table prepared with a blank sheet of butcher paper, have six to eight group members place their three objects in the center of the paper.
7. Ask each member to describe the objects they created/brought and why they chose them. When each person has shared, introduce the group portion of the project.
8. Collectively, you have all arrived on this island. You will now become a team whose job is to survive together. How will you each use the objects you brought for the group?
9. Decide together what your island will look like, what terrain it will have, what resources are available. Begin to create your island together, preparing to develop a plan to survive.
10. As each member engages and the group works together, ask questions to facilitate progress, address challenges, and promote dialogue.

Rationale

This directive is a group project that allows team building, assessment of group dynamics, and exploration of personal roles in a group. Furthermore, the limitation of the materials in the construction of the objects brought to the island presents an opportunity for problem solving. Discussing within the group of the objects brought and their meaning/importance helps individuals assert themselves independently before moving into the group problem-solving challenge.

Figure 6.27 is an image of the objects the survivors brought to the island with them. These have been sculpted from construction paper.

Figure 6.28 is a view of the island after constructed, complete with objects placed on it.

Personal Comments—22-Year-Old Female
Student of Professor Kagin

I thought that this exercise was incredibly fun. I felt like a little kid again, coming up with ideas in my imaginary games. The guided imagery was very relaxing, and the images that came to mind were definitely ones from movies I had seen and wanted to be a part of, so I used those to make up the beautiful cruise in my mind. Then, the horn did not alarm me too much, other than it awoke me from my nap in the sunlight. I did not panic when we were

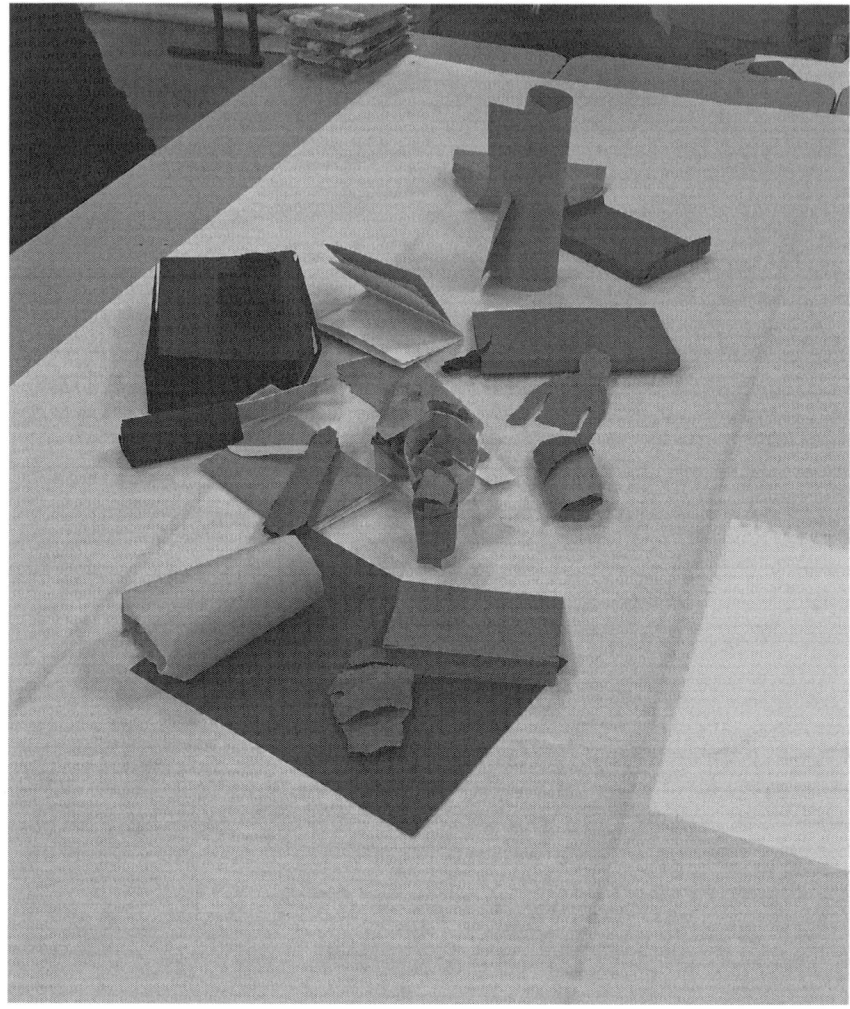

Figure 6.27 Survival on an Island

told there was something wrong or that we had to evacuate. I did prepare by gathering things that would keep me entertained and emotionally healthy, as well as trying to find a priest to hear my confession in case something were to happen. When I landed on the island, I distinctly remember being barefoot and really loving the way the sand and water felt on my feet. Then the next part, making our objects we brought with us was super annoying since we could not use anything but the paper to make the objects. Mine were subpar because when I am stuck doing things that I find annoying, I just try to get

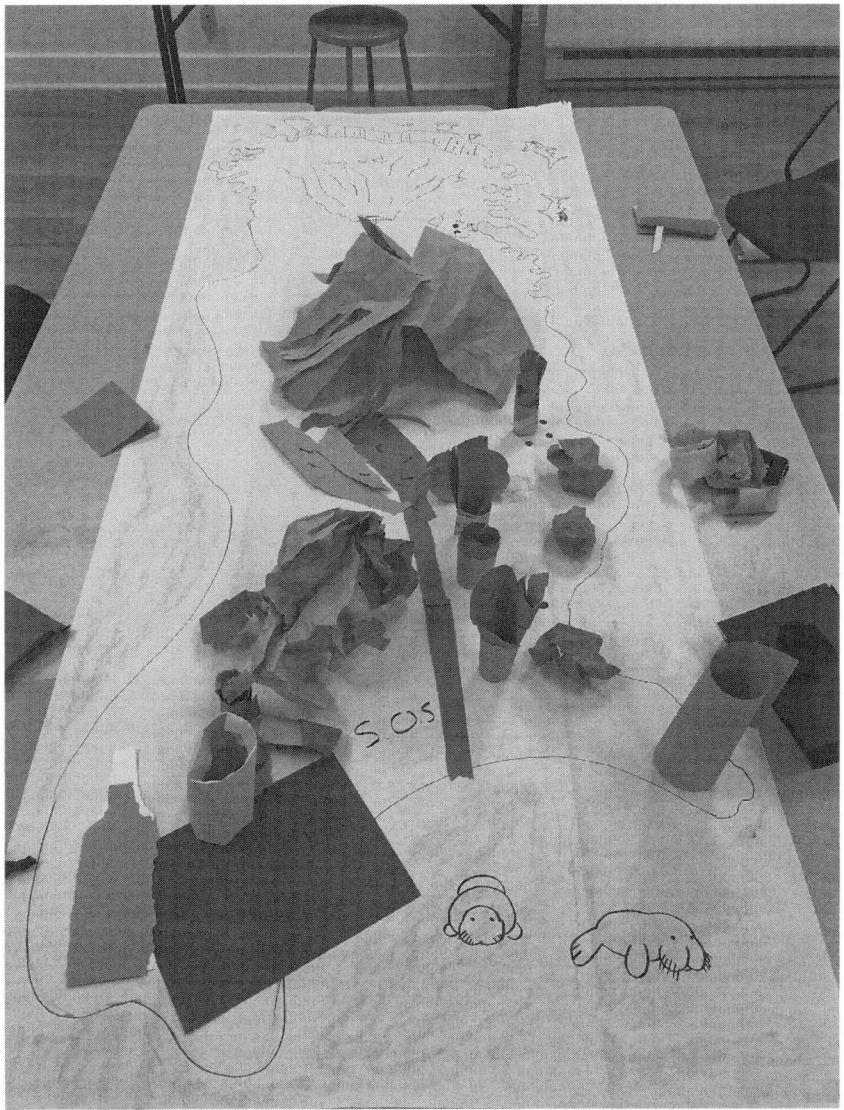

Figure 6.28 Survival on an Island

them done as fast as possible. When talking about what we brought, most people thought of food or survival related things. I brought a bottle of water to make sure I stayed hydrated until we could find another water source, but my camera and book were to keep my spirits high. I had a deep sense of trust as far as believing there would be someone who had brought some food or tools. I brought what I literally would have had with me on the cruise. I did not think of a tent or matches because I would not have had those with me. I figured the island would also have resources, and since the cruise ship knew we were having difficulties, I expected rescue to have been called and on their way. When we had to plan out the island, I did not want to call a lot of the shots, but I knew I wanted 3-D elements, so H.A. and I started making things with construction paper. I made the trees, which was interesting since I also did the trees on the last group mural we did last semester. But yes, I made the trees and brushes and included fruit on them. I also helped make the pond by the mountain and drew fish in there. When asked what I could contribute to the group's survival, I had to think back to camp. I was considered one of the best fire builders. I also knew how to set up tents the fastest. I have had a lot of experience working with what I have, so I had no doubt in my ability to make-shift things from sticks, vines, and whatever else I could find in nature, too. I also love to explore, so I was willing to do that for the group. When placed in the scenario that would determine the leader of the group, I could tell certain people really wanted the position. However, I also knew that certain personality types would perhaps not want to listen to other certain personality types in the room. I knew that everyone in the room seemed to get along well with me, but I waited, thought up a plan after looking at our layout, and then spoke. Everyone was talking over each other and not thinking through their plans, so I finally yelled "Everyone needs to calm down! We need to come up with a plan so we can work together towards a common goal. Right now, the most pressing thing is that we need food. So, I suggest that we kill one of the wild pigs, cook it and then come up with a way to make nets using vines so we can catch fish since the spears are not working." Then I delegated jobs to people. After we were fed, we needed to come up with a way to get off the island. Someone suggested a signal fire, to which I thought would be best to do after getting to the highest part of the island and scouting for sight of land, then building the fire on that side of the island so it would be seen more easily. Someone translated that as needing to build the fire on top of the mountain, so there was some debate about how that was going to waste energy. Then thankfully, Ashley suggested that we actually spend some time having fun together since everyone was so stressed. I agreed and suggested that we work during the daylight and then relax in the evenings with everyone. I think the most impressive thing that happened with the exercise is how we worked to do what was best for the whole group, not just ourselves or one other person in the group. I also felt like I went from not really being sure what to do and just doing something I knew would be useful to taking the leadership role because I figured it would be more beneficial for me to say something than everyone talking over one another. I felt a lot more confident in my own ideas and voice after people listened to me, too.*

Therapeutic Transition

It is intriguing to look at what this young lady chose to bring with her—water, camera, and book. She was confident others would bring survival tools they would all need. The water is life sustaining and also symbolically represents psychic energy. She has a great deal of positivity in her thinking but also relies on others to meet her needs. This is probably developmental, as she is young and in college, a time when exploration of the self is paramount and maintenance is left to parents or significant others. She obviously considers her situation temporary, as she will run out of water and battery power or electricity to power her camera (or film if it is not digital). Her leadership skills need to be further encouraged without them becoming control issues. How are they going to kill the pig? Encourage development of details in planning and having contingencies when the plan does not go the way expected.

Creativity Activation

Creativity is activated when the guided imagery begins to encourage visuals in the mind of the participant. From that point on, creativity builds through the creation of objects and the problem solving for media and tool limitations and further when the island itself must become a tangible image. As the group works to solve the challenges of survival and teamwork, the problem solving enhances the creative elements of this directive.

Adaptation

This initiative can be structured in several different ways. One is to give more structure and assign directives in some order such as how to designate organization and set priorities for the group. Another is to focus more on the group dynamics and ask who is to be in charge of what function such as housing, exploring, tool making, and so on. This is a powerful experience, and tensions may arise among the groups. If there are more than eight people, then there will need to be two islands. We have actually seen the islands go to war with each other! Intervention by the therapist or instructor may be necessary to get closure on any conflict before completing the initiative.

Initiative Twenty-Eight—The Bridge (Bridge the Opposites)

ETC—Kinesthetic/Sensory (K/S), Perceptual/Affective (P/A), and Cognitive/Symbolic (C/S)
MDV—High Complexity Unstructured Resistive (HCUR)

The symbolism of a bridge is used in our culture to represent many things. It also is a necessary component of our landscape and environment. The richness of the bridge in this initiative is used metaphorically to represent transformation of self from where the individual has been to where he or she is going.

Materials

Plasticine clay of a variety of colors

Directives

1. Create a form or symbol that represents where you are today.
2. Create a form or symbol that represents where you are going or want to be.
3. Create a bridge between the two forms you have created.
4. Create a form to represent yourself and place it somewhere on the bridge.
5. Process.

Rationale

The metaphor of the bridge is easily relatable, and the client can connect the idea of bringing two things together simply. A bridge takes you from one place to another, typically over an impassable area. Providing an opportunity for the client to concretely produce a visualization of movement helps them to see the potential for successfully achieving a goal.

Figure 6.29 shows an aerial view of two star-like forms in multicolored plasticine clay, connected by a thin white piece of clay representing a bridge. To the left side of the bridge is an oval multicolored form that represents the actual location of the woman in her journey.

Personal Comments—22-Year-Old Female
Student of Professor Kagin

Both where I am and where I want to be are not that far from each other. They looked similar, but one was bigger, more open . . . like a fuller version

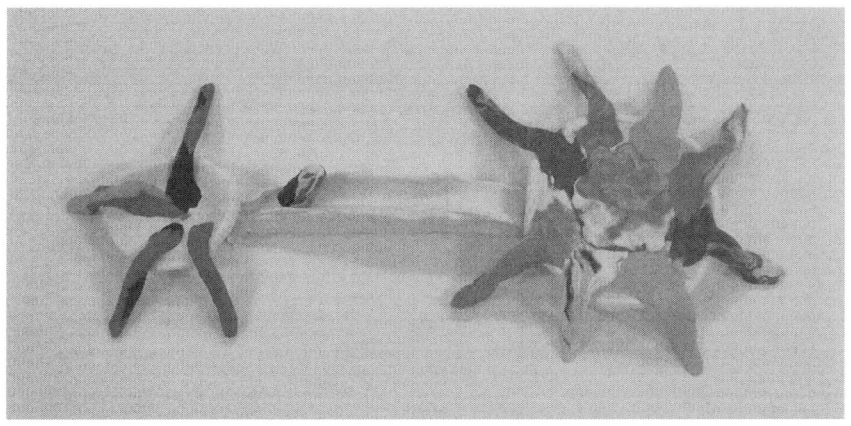

Figure 6.29 The Bridge (Bridge the Opposites)

of myself where I am now. The bridge is white, pure, straight and narrow, leading me to that fuller self. Where I am and where I want to be are touching the bridge, because I see my goal as achievable. I included white in the colors on the side of where I want to be, because the colors represent different aspects of myself but are more pure and light than where I am. Where I am going is a fuller version of self, represented with the white added. I am a vessel, and the colors pour out of me now and will then, too, when I reach where I want to be. I am on the bridge, close to where I am but moving forward to where I want to be.

Therapeutic Transition

This woman is secure in her present situation in life and appears confident and committed to her forward movement. The spilling out of the colors from self increases in the future self. Exploring more specific elements of self through the body-tracing initiative that represents real self and ideal self could be an additional clarification of what she seeks to pursue and would help to identify concrete steps toward fulfillment of this goal.

Figure 6.30 is a plasticine bridge featuring a brown base with a large black form and small red and green attachments on the left, connected to a blue bridge in the center and a white mound of clay on the right.

Personal Comments—22-Year-Old Female
Where I Am: It's not a physical place. My physical location means nothing. It's all about what's inside. The place I am in is all about my circumstances; here I have been placed, with these things I can't control. I knew that "the

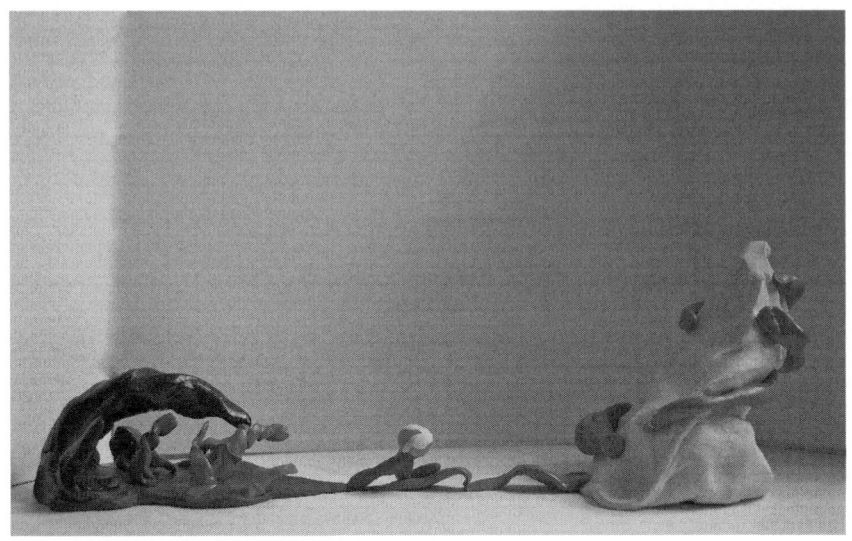

Figure 6.30 The Bridge (Bridge the Opposites)

place I am in" could not be a happy place. There are many unhappy elements of my life. I allowed each of my current unhappy elements to take form in a tendril. I formed each one, started from the back and moving forward, allowing their shape and color to be spontaneous.

The largest black tendril—my father.

The smaller black tendril—my brother.

Green tendrils—(1) money, (2) work, (3) stress and exhaustion relating to both. Together they form the longing to rest my body.

Red tendrils—(1) questioning God's presence, (2) lack of trust in others, (3) conflicting emotions toward my male best friend.

Together they form the theme of love and my questioning of how it exists.

These all came easily and quickly to me. I am no stranger to their presence in my life. They are always in the back of my mind.

Where I Want To Be: Again, it is not a physical place. More importantly, it's not a place that eliminates all of my problems. I imagine this place not to exist separate from the first place, but above it. Maybe that's why it became the form of a mountain. I don't need to get away from my problems. I don't want to erase them or have a perfect life. I just want to rise above it all. My struggles can be the base of the mountain, and I can climb it all to victory.

The blue clouds represent confidence, independence, helping others, and having friends I can trust and rely on. Together, these are all about loving myself, loving others, and trusting and accepting and receiving love from others.

Myself On The Bridge: I have my feet in both worlds. I constantly have my back turned to all the negativity, but nothing I can do can make it go away. All I can control is myself and how I respond to adversity.

Therapeutic Transition

This young woman is clearly struggling with male relationships at this time in her life. The size and overpowering element of the black tendril (father) shows the dominance this single relationship has at this point in her life. Her striving to move beyond her struggles is positive and should be nurtured. It would be good for her to perhaps explore this challenge in a battle drawing. Identifying and using archetype figures would shift some of the focus from self and allow the roles to become opportunities to express what she has not through the battle drawing. Furthermore, a battle could be drawn that would push back the tendrils from their approach to the bridge. Encouraging her confidence and desire to conquer the struggles by climbing to victory over them could be explored in guided imagery to the source.

Creativity Activation

Creativity is activated when the client creates a symbol of self and makes decisions about how to form the elements of this initiative. The bridge furthers the creativity as the metaphor but in a tangible form. This creativity helps to problem solve mobility and encourages movement.

Adaptation

One option is to change the media to a more resistive form and ask that the bridge be created out of wooden sticks and glue. This process would take more time and allows more reflection. The structure of the bridge would be analogous to the manner in which the person structures their life. Thus the problem solving becomes more important, as the individual must make a solid structure that stands and is functional. This reinforces the ability to move from one place in life to another.

References

Graves, S. (1994). *Expressions of Healing: Embracing the Process of Grief*. Hollywood, CA: Newcastle.

Jung, C. (1968). *Man and His Symbols*. New York, NY: Dell Publishing.

Kabat-Zinn, J. (2013). *Full Catastrophe Living: Using the Wisdom of Your Body and Mind to Face Stress, Pain, and Illness*. New York, NY: Random House.

Pearson, C. (1991). *Awakening the Heroes Within: Twelve Archetypes to Help Us Find Ourselves and Transform Our World*. New York, NY: Harper Collins.

Pearson, C. (1998). *The Hero Within: Six Archetypes We Live By*. New York, NY: Harper One.

Ronnberg, A. (Ed. in chief) and Martin, K. (Ed.) (2010). *The Book of Symbols: Reflections on Archetypal Images*. Cologne, Germany: Taschen.

Siegel, D. (2012). *Pocket Guide to Interpersonal Neurobiology: An Integrative Handbook of the Mind*. New York, NY: Norton and Company.

CHAPTER 7

Creativity and Its Role

Christa Kagin

Time and again I've noticed or seen or discovered how creativity activation brings a new way of thinking about a situation, a challenge, or a problem. Whether it be in the studio—when a student has painter's block or artist's block and the inability to find a way to discover the solution—or an opportunity for someone to explore a problem or a challenge or an emotion on a piece of paper or with the given materials. The physical challenge of being able to think creatively to solve small problems that seem unrelated to a larger problem opens up the mind, and the thought processes tap into a new way of thinking that allows for new ideas to come into view—a new way of expressing or thinking. Any time this happens, there is a response that is a change in emotion that happens and follows.

In this chapter, creativity is explored in three categories: data management, brain flow, and resolution. Within each category, special attention has been given to the manner in which the variables of the media dimensions and/or the process of the expressive therapies continuum affect three areas of our brain and mind—arousal, action, and homeostasis—and how these may result in the ongoing development of resiliency in an individual.

It has long been known that mindset alters physiological responses and can significantly enhance performance (a mother lifting a car off her toddler or an amazing act of superhuman prowess in some athletes). Today the term has become "zone hackers" (Kotler, 2014), wherein the ultimate "high" that is experienced at peak moments (the "zone") is actually derived from the brain (precortical transient hypofrontality) as it slows down and disengages from neurobiology and neurochemistry to deactivate higher cognitive functions. The ego function is bypassed! This has been found in any altered state, whether from narcotics, high-risk situations, or high levels of creative performance when endorphins are engulfing the body. An intuitive "voice" is also heard in what Jung (1968) described as perception from the unconscious. Intuition is now seen as a standard part of flow. Creativity also involves pattern recognition: how the brain "connects" things, thus yielding an output of dopamine, which in turn tightens focus. Alpha waves increase, which results in a calming of the system. All this helps the brain make connections between subconscious and conscious awareness and causes an increase in theta waves, which are responsible for intuition and idea generation (Thompson-Schill et al., 2009).

Data Management, Brain Flow, and Resolution

Data Management

Creativity activation is a critical component to what we are looking at in the Expressive Therapies Continuum (ETC). We believe it is important to give people the opportunity to see and experience challenges and struggles in new ways. These activities bring about the activation of thought and response and problem solving that brings into play a new idea. For example, when I have students who are stuck on a project or assignment, I may give them three or four creativity exercises, or I may give them 10 exercises, and then I tell them that this is their homework that they must complete before they are able to go back to their project. Even if they get an idea along the way, they have to write that idea down or do a quick thumbnail and then return to the creativity exercises. Sometimes just being given the challenge of having to see something in a new way will open our eyes to possibilities because it changes our focus and it changes our attitude, and it often changes our emotions and assists in reaching a flow state.

Creativity Exercises

One of the tasks that I give students is to copy a child's drawing. I allow them to get the drawing off of the internet or find something that they have seen or maybe a drawing from a family member or from their own childhood. The direction on this creativity exercise is to copy the original and make changes as they come to mind such as emphasizing a line, enlarging a shape, changing a color. Students are asked to consider potential reasons for these changes. Did they recall a memory? Did it elicit an emotional response? Copying and changing the drawing is an important component of the assignment because it simplifies the idea that something must be a particular way and notes an awareness of new information over time. One of the struggles that we have in life when we are facing challenges is the mentality that things must be a certain way. When we focus on the act of copying something that doesn't necessarily meet all of the criteria for being a perfectly drawn house or a perfectly formed human figure or a dog, the drawing copy seems fun, light, and lively. That activity and that interaction opens us up into a little bit of laughter and a little bit of joy and definitely spontaneity. Our minds begin to think about it, and when we think about a child's drawing of a dog with a funny body, it makes us laugh. Then we begin to think about it, and we think *Well, what if I did this?* or *What if I did that to it?* and before you know it we have begun to make a series of lines or marks or ideas that have come from something that was very simple. Maybe your creation is just a series of shapes, but it's the way that the lines have been connected or related, or maybe it's the way that color has been used in an unexpected way that makes the new drawing inventive. Any of these things that a child is going to use in an uninhibited way helps to free us from our own inhibitions. This freedom helps us to see things as fresh and new. This activity is very similar to what happens in the creativity activation in our own art therapy projects. What we are doing here is taking information that has been stored and putting it in a new context that brings about a new awareness of its meaning or use. This is a form of problem solving we use every day without realizing we are seeding a creative experience.

A second creativity exercise is to make marks on a page with a single tool, using graphite or ink. Draw without thinking about the marks. Draw until you feel that you are finished. Once you reach that point, choose another medium, preferably one of color, and add to the original drawing. Consider what it felt like to make marks freely without restrictions or expectations. Observe how your hand moves. Are you tight and controlled or loose and free? Did you vary your marks, or are they similar across the page and vary only in direction? How did it change when you added color? Were you hesitant to add the color? What was the difference in how it felt from the beginning to the end? This exercise is a good example of using the Kinesthetic/Sensory (K/S) level and allowing the properties of the media to give new information and awareness to the task. For the larger relationship to the studio assignment, I ask, "How can you use this knowledge and apply it to your project?"

Changing perspective is another direction to take. Draw something from a new angle; for example, turn the teacup upside down or draw something sitting on the edge of a table while you sit on the floor. This change in observation provides new information about the object and makes us realize there are many dimensions to an object, which can translate also to an idea or thought. Perhaps the new perspective makes the object, which at first seems simple, much more interesting and provocative.

Recollection of memories can elicit great imagery for drawing and free expression but needs to be pushed further for the creativity to be fully activated. The student is told to recall a memory from childhood and then draw three things that are seen in the mind while recalling this event on separate pieces of paper. Drawing these objects is the first step, and they are to be drawn simply as objects on the page. Once completed, put the drawings beside each other and look at these objects again. The student is then prompted to draw what the three objects conjure up in his or her mind as seen together. This is often very different than the original memory and thus propels the mind into associating the objects in a new way. In essence what is being done is that new neural pathways are being created. For example, one student recalled a birthday party at which she got a tricycle. Her three objects drawn were a party hat, a balloon, and the tricycle. The drawing born from these three objects was an elaborate flying machine with pedals! She became excited during this process, thus arousal occurred that motivated an entirely new idea. A new vitality for approaching the original homework assignment was produced by this creative flow, giving it a new valence of importance and motivation.

Using a different medium than ink or graphite, the student is instructed to write a paragraph about the most beautiful moment in her life or the most beautiful thing she has ever seen. Then assign the experience a color that represents that beauty. Leave it for a period of time, then return to it later and "create something." The responses have ranged from drawings to collage and embellished objects in sculptural form. They are then given the following to ponder:

To be creative, you need to step outside of yourself, see things again for the first time, listen to life's sounds, become mesmerized by the details, experience the beauty around you in unexpected places. To do this, you need to define beauty in a wholeness, encompassing what can be seen and what cannot. You must embrace all that becomes evident to you and prepare to respond . . . freely, uninhibited. You must actively seek.

The above exercises translate from the studio classroom to the art therapy room. While we may not ask a client to copy a child's drawing or the client may be a child himself, we will be using the same concept of triggering change through creativity by means of offering opportunities to create based on prompts that we provide. The student may have copied a child's drawing, but we may even use images of other drawings in a session to encourage dialogue and to release inhibitions that clients have about making art. To simplify an image or a challenge into only a few lines or nonlocal colors inspires a new thought and a new response. If a tree should be green but is painted purple, how then does that relate to our expectations in life? This introduction of creativity exercises has its place in education but also in daily life. As art therapists, we teach our clients through exposures to art materials that things can be changed and even seen differently and that we are not restricted to what we have always thought or always known.

Brain Flow

Kotler (2014, p. viii) defines flow as an "optimal state of consciousness where we feel our best and perform our best. It is also a strange state of consciousness." He goes on:

> Concentration becomes so laser focused that everything else falls away. Action and awareness merge. Our sense of self and our sense of self-consciousness completely disappear. Time dilates—meaning it slows down like the freeze frame of a car crash or speeds up and five hours pass by in five minutes. And throughout, all aspects of performance are incredibly heightened and that includes creative performance.

We are adopting Kotler's definition for purposes of our operational definition of flow. Another example of this is the experience that has been described as "ecstasy" by artists when they are at the peak of their creation. Ecstasy becomes an altered state of mind, which Kotler refers to as the zone and Mihaly Csikszentmihalyi calls ecstasy (Csikszentmihalyi, 2008).

Resonance and Resolution

In Kagin and Lusebrink's article on the Expressive Therapies Continuum (1978), creativity was the fourth level of the continuum but present in all the levels to some degree. At the Kinesthetic level, the discovery of resonance with the media can lead to an intensified experience with the materials that are "new" to the individual. At the Perceptual level, new form is created as sensorimotor entrainment gives way to awareness of creating figure–ground relationships. Information is processed at the cognitive/symbolic level that was unknown to the creator prior to the process. Creativity is, indeed, inherent and necessary in development.

We know that when this experience we call creativity is activated, we experience pleasure. Endorphins are released in the body, which allows reduction of stress and counters negative perceptions. We become open to new information and ideas, thus altering the neural pattern previously associated with the awareness and factual data being explored (Siegel, 2012).

Exploring the Self through Creativity

Propensity toward creativity is inherent in all people. While it has often been associated with genius (Albert Einstein, Benjamin Franklin, Leonardo da Vinci, Pablo Picasso), it is not limited to genius. Creativity is in fact something that can be fostered and experienced in each person given the right circumstances and stimuli. The capacity to tap into elements of thinking, doing, and processing stimulated by creative actions encourages change.

The exploration of the self through visual media is a creative endeavor. It takes a person on a journey, requiring thought, challenge, and response to a variety of experiences in life, prompts, and stimuli that facilitate an activation of creativity. To define creativity today is not easy. The scientific world has a definition and varying ideas of what creativity is and how it develops and is manifested. Mental health practitioners have their own ideas about creativity's role in the treatment of a client. Art educators have an understanding of what they believe to be creativity and creative responses to prompts in the classroom. Artists themselves define creativity in a more unique way than the scientific definition. These varying viewpoints can cause confusion: What is creativity, and how do you define it? Why is it important? What can it do? While the answers to these questions are not black and white, exploring them will hopefully help the reader to understand why we have identified creativity activation following each initiative and why we value its role in the healing process. For purposes of an operational definition, we have adopted the brain flow information and refer to how creativity can be activated after each initiative. It should also be noted that often, the use of visual breathing precedes the project as a means of putting the student or client into a more relaxed state before the arousal that occurs using the materials.

Science and Creativity

Scientific research is asking many questions about creativity. Some define it as a process by which people become aware of problems or challenges or even ideas and knowledgeable facts, and then by defining the problem and searching out solutions, they can communicate discoveries and answers to the original problem identified (Torrance, 1965). This definition is slightly different than the practical and spontaneous responses we see in the art therapy session or the classroom.

This exploration and research into the cognitive science of the brain's ability to solve problems, think, and process information, though it is helpful to us as it provides validity to the topic of creativity, also creates a polarity between the applications of science and art that serves as a kind of continuum from the more explicit scientific method to the spontaneous expression in flow. This is significant because creativity has found its way into the mainstream of business, education, treatment, and research.

Education and Creativity

In education, creativity is defined more as a means by which imagination is activated and then produces results through application to a problem (Robinson, 2006). This distinction embodies more of the spontaneity that we seek to foster and manifest through art therapy initiatives, as imagination can be activated and explored without a predetermined outcome. For example, if I am doing an assessment and use the House—Tree—Person projective (Jolles, 1971), I expect that the house will look like a house or housing unit. But if I ask a client to create a self-portrait and they paint all yellow with a black spot in the middle, this is acceptable and progressive, as they have painted and responded. However, in a classroom with the same prompt to create a self portrait this would be considered wrong because there would be the expectation that the portrait look like a face. For us, the goal is not the beauty or aesthetic of the end product but rather about the process of the creative flow itself and how the client can reflect back upon the response and experience something new or analyze something in a productive manner for growth. We use the product as both a catalyst and also a concrete example of success. In education, solving problems employs specific research-based techniques to foster learning through creative means including questions, brainstorming, and action-centered play (puppets, role-play, objects; Chávez-Eakle, 2010). Using both convergent and divergent thinking, it allows students to be able to visualize problems, think about them anew, and even create with new insight, utilizing external and internal response (Chávez-Eakle, 2010). This is exactly the power of the art directives to facilitate specific paths that can focus a client on a particular challenge but also can be used without deeply therapeutic processing and can aid students in their ability to face challenges, work in groups, interact with peers, and find new ways to approach learning. This is useful for the educator as a means of creating goals for the classroom, for individuals, and for learning outcomes. Preparing for the utilization of initiatives in the classroom with a specific topic or issue as focus could put the students in place to work and respond but also develop an understanding collectively and individually. For example, the use of the persona masks as part of a group activity could provide insight into social activity and comfort with peers by allowing students to recognize we may have more than one way of feeling in a group and more than one way of behaving in a group, and peers do as well. Creating two masks of "conflicting sides of self in groups" (or the playground, classroom, group project, or other) would facilitate a discussion, engage students in thinking about their multifaceted personalities, and activate an animated role-play wherein students could "safely" say or act out roles behind a mask and peers could relate. This activity would provide insights for the teacher regarding the emotional states of his/her students and also be informative for the development of teams, projects, and classroom management.

Recognizing that there is more than one side to self and one's reactions can be transformative for students who have vacillating emotions and do not understand that others also experience this. This creative approach to groups could help students to adapt to their classroom spaces, as creative thinking fosters new understanding and problem solving, thereby transforming the experience into one of positivity and awareness. Aiding students (children and adolescents) through the use of creativity-activating projects could have impacts far beyond the scope of a single lesson or classroom, even into the family environment and extracurricular activities (Chávez-Eakle, 2010).

In a similar way, Survival on an Island could be used in the classroom for team development, creative problem solving, and outcome goals. The island is metaphorically the classroom, and students "survive" together. Revisiting the island during the year with objects students have created, adapted, or traded could be a great on-going project application for cohesion and self-esteem. Journals could be kept for reflection and application of the island metaphor to the classroom and other learning. This would foster creativity on a long-term basis for a measurable impact on learning throughout the school year. This initiative is effective for group dynamics, problem solving, identification of strengths and weaknesses, membership in a group, and altruistic experiences. The implications and possibilities are nearly endless with this encouragement of creativity activation.

Art and Creativity

Artists will say about themselves that creativity is necessary and that it ebbs and flows, producing different kinds of work and both successes and failures. Most will also acknowledge the flow experience in which time stands still and ideas resonate seamlessly. The creative process then can be distinguished as separate from a product that can be described as creative. How is this distinction made? Why is it even necessary?

Thinking patterns are one of the greatest impacts on success and failure. Successful thinking can create positive results and motivate someone to work and achieve goals and make changes. Thinking patterns that are negative, however, or that have cyclical elements that can be limiting or restrictive in one's ability to process information correctly or make changes, can lead to failure. Asking questions, requiring actions, and processing outcomes can change these thinking patterns. Sometimes, while the desire may be there to make changes, the ability to do so is lacking. When a person has thought the same way for years and never been challenged to think about something in a new way, change is nearly impossible. This is how art therapy can provide insights but also why understanding creativity and its role in the therapeutic process can help to bring about more success and new neural patterns, resulting in new thoughts.

The first step is to recognize the pattern or problem. Art, because it is outside of self, allows an opportunity for this to take place. Reflecting on the product produced and the many aspects of the directives and responses can bring insight to a pattern and encourage the client to see the need for change and even ways to change. These responses are produced when creativity is activated. Without being pushed into these art actions, it is unlikely that a person would conjure up tasks or questions to address thinking patterns or issues they are facing. However, with the mere act of being given the directives and materials to complete the steps, clients must begin a new way of thinking that promotes an ability to problem solve. The more exposure and practice of creating visual responses to prompts takes place, the more the mind begins to think differently and solve in new ways. This is the creativity. The therapist then has the opportunity to go or push with the client to explore the issues or challenges by means of the product. Emphasizing the creativity is encouraging and informative. To know that you have the means to discover new ways of thinking about or responding to situations provides a hopeful and uplifting emotional state. Change is possible. Insight is not just for other people. Action produces results.

When we approach thinking, it is through a self-contained canon that is activated without intention or focus. Our order of thoughts comes from the historical blueprints written into our cortex and amygdala from our experiences. For comfort or survival, we have developed responses and sequences of thoughts that have established our behavioral reactions and challenges, leaving us where we are today. We do not naturally just add a new way of thinking or processing into this bank of emotional outlines and acquire new responses. We must recognize and access these standards of thinking and, by becoming aware of them, explore how to insert new information. The application of creativity here, inspired by external stimuli, can aid the insertion of new ideas to impregnate the current system of principles in the thought pattern. How can this be so?

Referring to Chapter 6 and the initiative of the Word, this idea of seeing things anew from the interpretation of response to words and application to self is evident. *This made me aware of how little control I have over certain things I'm given in life (words) but also made me aware of how much control I still have over what I do with those words. . . . This forced me to see words not so much for what they are, but for whatever meaning I assigned to them. Instead of just seeing them at face value, I gave them a context in which to be seen* (see Personal Comments for Initiative Twelve). The external stimuli were the directives and the materials provided to create the initiative. The new ideas of understanding how the words can become more than what they are on their own, before projection, allows the client to see that our responses can often be inhibitors to truth and antagonists to self and relationships. It is through the free association (current connections) and forced interactions with words (separate from self, not chosen) that the creativity is activated and applied. This is similar to the problem-solving collage (Chapter 6), which requires parts of a problem (current connections and thinking) to be transformed into discrete shapes and then arranged into an aesthetic composition. Extracting meaning after originating the shapes and then arranging them into an intentional structure promotes distance and reflection. Examination of the key then allows association of the shapes to reinstate meaning. Creativity applied in the beginning stages precipitates new connections and thus a creative way of viewing and approaching the problem. The way clients create and assign shapes is often stimulating in the processing, as they can creatively relate concepts, such as the free shapes becoming the most challenging parts of the issue to identify, and thus that shape isn't identifiable by a name either. What then can we do but see it relationally to other shapes? We have reframed the problem. This creativity was born from the product, while creativity in the invention of the shapes is in the process. Because this produces alternatives to original problems, change is generated from the activated creativity.

Artists create works of art that allow us to see things as they are, such as in a Dutch still life, or as the artist wants us to see them from a new perspective, such as in Georgia O'Keefe's close-ups of flowers, or even in brand new ways, such as Picasso's cubist works. All of these have an intentional view put forth from the artist. However, they also have the way we explore, understand, and internalize them that makes them unique. Artists help us see things in new, fresh ways so our eyes can translate knowledge anew. Changing a color or a line or the materiality or the scale of an object can impact everything about the way we think and engage with the object. This is the same process by which the client changes his/her own perspective of elements within life, thereby seeing them freshly. The manipulation of the art materials activates the kinesthetic sensory responses, activating the perceptual and affective sensors, resulting in cognitive and symbolic understanding. Looking at art and learning about art is transformative, but creating art enlivens a deeper awareness and meaning, which, in the case of the ETC-MDV, cultivates change.

To bring something into being or to birth an idea that transforms something and/or causes its creation is creativity. Thoughts can promote action, and action can promote thought. Adding any word or material to the equation impacts the outcome. Asking and answering questions, exploring options, or looking can all change a response. So, if a client was to be given a prompt, asked a question, offered materials, and expected to problem solve for the answer, each step would ignite a different action or thought and thus birth a creative response. When creativity activation happens for individuals can be different, but it is often at similar times during the problem-solving process. When the thinking begins to answer the prompt, whether that be "paint your best day" or "make something with this clay," the materials and words initiate the response, and actions are connected. Thoughts can promote actions, and actions can promote thoughts. The opening in the perceived obstacle being faced is where the creativity seed begins to grow. Is that in thinking about the day, or is that in the materiality of paint or clay? Is that in the action of seeing a lump of clay and holding it to begin shaping it? Is it in the connection of the physical response and the mental response? Wherever it may be found, the seed is quickly nourished by thought and action, and the choices begin to be made, which each impact the other. Creativity grows here and promotes discovery, each leaf being new possibilities or even challenges, but connected to creativity and therefore nurtured by the new life that is the response. Thoughts and actions follow, and eyes see new or surprising creations. Symbolic connections are made, new insights become perceptible, and whether fully understood or only acknowledged, these beget the potential for transformation and/or invention. Therein the seed has produced life, not only in the creativity that has been activated but in the sense of being alive that comes from being able to look at, engage in, and solve a problem. A victory, though small (shaping clay into a regressive form or painting a blue sky with a yellow sun) can impact the sense of accomplishment, hope, and also self.

When Dr. Ken Robinson stated that "creativity is as important in education now as literacy" he was elevating the significance of creativity to the learning environment. For us, we know that creativity is part of living and should be fostered in children as well as adults because it aids in growth and progress and understanding. Creativity increases the vitality in tasks and the ability to problem solve and act. If this is not fostered and it thus could then be lost, the challenge of reintroducing it to adults, the act of being creative and thinking about how to do things without fear of failure, then people can become crippled (Robinson, 2006). In art therapy, product is not the goal, but what happens during the process on the way to the product transforms the client. This is why through the initiatives, we think it is important for the practitioner to consider and encourage creativity, to be aware of it and its propensity for activating awareness and healing. These initiatives explore many aspects of experiencing life, through sound and a variety of media, movement, touch, and visuals. This is important to learning and thinking. As Robinson further stated, "We think about the world in all the ways that we experience it. We think visually, we think in sound, we think kinesthetically. We think in abstract terms, we think in movement" (2006). This thinking can be nurtured through art therapy and its initiatives. More than nurturing it, though, art therapy can arouse this thinking through the creativity activated by *doing* the creating. Process therefore helps to produce something original to that moment, to that client, to that student, something brand new through addressing the prompt (problem—challenge) to concentrate on the issue (problem—behavior—conflict) to find a solution through *creation*.

In recent years, a decrease in creativity has been noted in a study by Kyung Hee Kim (2011), producing concern for the limitations this could potentially generate and the long-term implications of this decrease. In a *Newsweek* article, Bronson and Merryman (2010) presented this information with the title "The Creativity Crisis," creating a red flag in a mainstream publication and citing the weight of this research (Bronson and Merryman, 2010). With a decline in creativity scores, as measured by Torrance Tests of Creative Thinking (TTCT), there is a more significant need for creativity to be a focus in wellness and mental health and also education. As the original Torrance (and now Garnet Miller) studies have shown, creativity scores were a better indicator of lifetime creativity than IQ scores were (Bronson and Merryman, 2010). We can translate this into applicable knowledge for the practitioner or educator using the foundation of the ETC-MDV and asserting the importance of this framework into the session or the classroom for the student/client. If we know that creativity can be activated and nurtured, then we have an opportunity to utilize the arts to reintroduce this potential in people. As Winnicott identified, meaning of life and awareness of self are impacted by the act of creativity (1971).

Referencing the creativity activation in each of the initiatives, this clinical guide offers not only an understanding of the Expressive Therapies Continuum and the Media Dimension Variables related to specific art therapy initiatives, but it also highlights how the implementation of the directives in each can activate and foster creative responses. This important inclusion empowers the practitioner or educator to apply knowledge of the ETC-MDV to other initiatives, activities, or projects with the additional goal of inspiring and activating creativity for the betterment of the client, student, or group. In a time when creativity scores are down for America (Kim, 2011), this insight could not be more useful.

Applying the ETC-MDV to the Science, Technology, Engineering, Art, and Mathematics (S.T.E.A.M.) Approach to Education

Science, technology, engineering, and math (STEM) have been at the core of education and innovation for several years. Recently, however, the addition of art has been accelerating rapidly, yielding the STEAM emphasis, in which industries are being encouraged to hire artists to further innovation. Many if not all of our initiatives can be adapted to the classroom from K through 12. Integration is the foundation of STEAM from body motion, visual perception, cognitive problem solving, and creative use of materials and processes. How does mathematics relate to life, building, painting, technology, and career choices? STEAM focuses on left- and right-brain development—how to do something differently with the same or better outcome.

Wherein we know that creating art has a propensity toward encouraging creativity, we think that the application of the initiatives and even the underlying knowledge and understanding that comes from the initiatives found within this book could aid and propel education within STEAM movements and programs. As we outlined in the creativity section, there is an element of creativity that is naturally fostered in the scientific method of finding a problem, seeking solutions, trying those solutions, finding out what fails and what successes are, and then rethinking it until you find the result. This is definitely a method that students are learning through the STEAM programs. We also understand that the process of thinking about technology and design of technology must be born from creative thinking and problem solving. There are storyboards and iterations pinned up around offices and think tanks where people are trying to problem solve again. In the use of problem solving as a way to think about how to apply new ideas to technology and integrate knowledge that already exists but also to create a catalyst to move it forward in such examples as this, some are using art and some are not. However, it is the belief of these authors that the use of art in situations in STEM or STEAM programs will help to foster a new way of working and a new way of problem solving that will move us even further forward into the 21st century. As we looked at our initiatives and thought about them in terms of education, in terms of time, in terms of technology and math, we considered adaptations for them. The following small sections outline some of those applications by which we think educators can apply these initiatives and these concepts to learning within a STEAM program. Here are some suggestions for use of our initiatives in STEAM education.

From Scribble Chase—Chapter 4
A body in motion stays in motion. Perception is both pathway and figure–ground relationships. Angles are entirely different from curvilinear forms, not only kinesthetically but in development of thinking as well. Social psychology and interpersonal relationships with people and cultures may also be explored. What happens when conflict occurs or roadblocks are put up? Would children and adults from different cultures behave differently with these directives? Why?

It is well known that graphic development follows a pattern whether the child lives in China, Africa, or the United States. Visual constructs also appear to be a universal language. How can we use this knowledge with our children? What can we teach them, and what can they discover?

From Expressions in Movement and Sound—Chapter 4
Explore how sound influences movement and visual expression. Would there be a difference if this initiative began with sound and instruments and then was translated visually? Why? Exploration of different parts of the brain would explain this phenomenon. Mathematically, would beat and rhythm affect movement, heart rate, and brain waves?

Media Properties—Chapter 4
This is a great introduction to the practical use of chemistry, volume, and physics, as well as mathematics and engineering. How much quantity or boundary is needed to initiate a creative response? Also ask the class to think of other materials that could be added to this exercise.

Body Tracing—Chapter 5
Teaching children about anatomy and why they feel and move the way they do can be very well illustrated by the body tracing. One body can be done as directed (the ideal self), and the real self can be assisted by an anatomical template to be put over the drawing. This could be exciting, as the meaning of different colors can be discussed as they relate to organs, muscular system, and so forth. At the same time, a lesson in chakras can be introduced. This blends information from both Western and Eastern cultures and integrates science with spirituality.

Guided Imagery—Chapter 6
The guided imagery initiatives are only a few examples of the many available for the teacher to use. Studies in mythology and anthropology may then be introduced. In addition, adaptation of guided imagery scripts could be a preparatory exercise for commencing a new project such as constructing a tower out of cardboard. Rather than giving directions on how to construct a tower, the student is taken to an alpha state activation place in which they imagine walking in a beautiful setting, where they encounter a tower made of cardboard. Look at it and explore how it is put together, how tall it is, and what shape it is. Then gather the students to discuss their various images and decide how to make their structure.

Box Self—Chapter 6
The box self initiative is, indeed, confined to the rectangular or square properties of "box." Here a lesson in geometry could enhance their understanding of the complexity (and simplicity) of the form that is being used to describe their inner and outer selves, melding mathematics to psychology.

Bridge—Chapter 6
The bridge initiative is a study in transition and transformation; therefore, it introduces complexities in psychology. The bridge is also a feat of engineering, dealing with the complexity of physics to span a piece of geography. Here, again, is an opportunity to broaden the students' thinking and perception of the integration of parts to the whole and the connectivity of which we may all be aware.

As is evident here, application of these initiatives can easily be inspiration for learning in the classroom, no matter the educational focus. The previously listed suggestions are just the beginning for the creative educator who seeks to always be learning and striving for better facilitation and better outcomes in the classroom. Encouraging creativity in students will certainly impact education from this point forward, aiding problem solving, teamwork, and leadership, as well as increasing self-awareness, making all-around more resilient students.

Life is entirely unthinkable without any of the creative arts, and they're all a continuum—the force in question is creativity, not its mode of expression.

John Darnielle, quoted in Spoerl (2012)

Conclusion

Creativity is not just a word to describe an action seen in young children who paint or draw or build castles in the sand. It is not an explanation for the gifted individual's abilities or the genius's works produced. It is not limited to science or math or music or art. It is not something that some people have and others do not (though what people do to cultivate it with their intelligence varies greatly). Creativity can be a small seedling planted, nurtured, and harvested, and, rather than decreasing, it could become the most significant gross national product in America. The importance we place on creativity and the manner in which we strive to encourage it has lasting impact beyond the social studies project, beyond the therapy session, and beyond the horizon we can see.

References

Bronson, P. and Merryman, A. (2010, July 10). The Creativity Crisis. *Newsweek*. Retrieved from http://www.newsweek.com/creativity-crisis-74665

Chávez-Eakle, R.A. (2010, Spring). *The Relevance of Creativity in Education*. The Johns Hopkins University New Horizons for Learning. Retrieved from http://education.jhu.edu/PD/newhorizons/Journals/spring2010/therelevanceofcreativityineducation/

Csikszentmihalyi, M. (2008, February). *Mihaly Csikszentmihalyi: Flow, the Secret of Happiness*. [Video file]. Retrieved from https://www.ted.com/talks/mihaly_csikszentmihalyi_on_flow?language=en

Jolles, I. (1971). *A Catalog for the Qualitative Interpretation of the House-Tree-Person (H-T-P)*. Los Angeles, CA: Western Psychological Services.

Jung, C. (1968). *Man and His Symbols*. New York, NY: Dell Publishing.

Kagin, S. and Lusebrink, V. (1978) The expressive therapies continuum. *Art Psychotherapy*, 5, 171–180.

Kim, K.H. (2011). The creativity crisis: The decrease in creative thinking scores on the Torrance tests of creative thinking. *Creativity Research Journal*, 23 (4), 285–295. doi:10.1080/10400419.2011.627805

Kotler, S. (2014). *The Rise of Superman: Decoding the Science of Ultimate Human Performance*. Boston & New York: New Harvest Houghton Mifflin Harcourt.

Robinson, K. (2006, June). *Ken Robinson: Do Schools Kill Creativity?* [Video file]. Retrieved from https://www.ted.com/talks/ken_robinson_says_schools_kill_creativity/transcript?language=en

Siegel, D. (2012). *Pocket Guide to Interpersonal Neurobiology: An Integrative Handbook of the Mind*. New York, NY: Norton and Company.

Spoerl, S. (2012, October 9). *Just Stay Alive: An interview with John Darnielle of the Mountain Goats*. [Steven Spoerl]. Retrieved from http://www.popmatters.com/feature/163980-heretic-pride-an-interview-with-john-darnielle/

Thompson-Schill, S., Ramscar, M. and Chrysikou, E. (2009). Cognition without control: When a little frontal cortex goes a long way. *Current Directions in Psychological Science*, 18, 259–263.

Torrance, P.E. (1965). Scientific views of creativity and factors affecting its growth. *Daedalus*, 94 (3), 663–681. Retrieved from https://www.jstor.org/stable/20026936

Winnicott, D.W. (1971). *Playing and Reality*. London: Tavistock Publications.

Appendix 1

Additional References

Arnheim, R. (1974). *Art and Visual Perception: A Psychology of the Creative Eye.* Berkeley, CA: University of California Press.

Barron, F.X. (1955). The disposition toward originality. *Journal of Abnormal Social Psychology*, 51, 478–485.

Barron, F.X. and Harrington, D.M. (1981) Creativity, intelligence, and personality. *Annual Review of Psychology*, 32, 439–476.

Cutraro, J. (2012). *How Creativity Powers Science.* Student Science. Retrieved from https://student.societyforscience.org/article/how-creativity-powers-science.

Edwards, D. (2008). *Artscience: Creativity in the Post Google Generation.* Cambridge, MA: Harvard University Press.

Eysenck, H.J. (1995). *Genius: The Natural History of Creativity.* New York, NY: Cambridge University Press.

Fasko, Jr., D. (2000–2001). Education and creativity. *Creativity Research Journal*, 13 (3 & 4), 317–327. Retrieved from www.valialoutrianaki.com/uploads/1/3/4/7/13471246/educ_creativity.pdf.

Fischer, E. (2010). *The Necessity of Art.* London & New York: Verso.

Franken, R.E. (1993). Curiosity, exploratory behavior, play, sensation seeking, and creativity. In *Human Motivation* (3rd ed.; chapter 12). New York: Brooks/Cole.

Greene, M. (2001). *Variation on a Blue Guitar: The Lincoln Center Institute Lectures on Aesthetic Education.* New York: Teachers College Press.

Guilford, J. (1965). A psychometric approach to creativity. In Anderson, H. (ed.), *Creativity in Childhood and Adolescence.* Palo Alto, CA: Science and Behavior Books, Inc.

Junge, M. (1994). *The History of Art Therapy in the United States*. Mundelin, IL: American Art Therapy Association.

Kelly, G. (1955). *The Psychology of Personal Constructs* (2 vols.). New York: Norton.

Pappano, L. (2014, February 5). Learning to think outside the box: Creativity becomes an academic discipline. *The New York Times*. Retrieved from http://www.nytimes.com/2014/02/09/education/edlife/creativity-becomes-an-academic-discipline.html?_r=1.

Rubin, J.A. (2010). *Introduction to Art Therapy: Sources and Resources*. New York, NY: Routledge.

Seelig, T. (2012). *InGenius, a Crash Course on Creativity*. New York, NY: HarperCollins.

Stites, R. (1970). *The Sublimations of Leonardo da Vinci*. Washington: Smithsonian Institution Press.

Appendix 2

Resources

American Dance Therapy Association. http://www.adta.org

American Music Therapy Association. http://www.musictherapy.org

Association for Play Therapy. http://a4pt.org

Expressive Media Inc. http://www.expressivemedia.org

International Expressive Arts Therapies Association. http://www.ieata.org

International Phototherapy Association—IPTA. http://www.jmll.co.jp/pta

National Association for Poetry Therapy. http://www.poetrytherapy.org

National Coalition of Creative Arts Therapies Associations. http://www.nccata.org

North American Drama Therapy Association. http://www.nadta.org

Index

12 Archetypes initiative 126–9

acceptance 71
adaptability 25
affective variable 13
ambiguity
    clarity vs. 46
    problem solving and 75
    tolerance for 51–2, 59, 70
American Art Therapy Association 3, 5
American Society of Psychopathology of Expression 4
anima and animus 130
archetypes 126–9
art
    classifying projects 10
    creativity and 167–71
    as therapy 3, 6
art behavior reinforcement group 10–11
art therapy 46, 170–1
assessment instrument 77
Ault, Bob 5

balance 46
Battle Drawing initiative 134–6
behavior boundaries 9
beta frequencies 16
body awareness/image
    difficulty in 32–3
    group work on 11
    inner feelings and 118
Body Tracing initiative 118–20, 173
Book of Symbols (Ronnberg) 98
boundaries and cognition 19–20
Box Self initiative 59, 115–17, 174
brain flow 163
brainwave entrainment (BWE) 16
Bridge initiative 154–7, 174
bridges, creativity activation 157
bridges, symbolism of 154
Bronson, P. 171
Bulletin of Art Therapy (journal) 3

Caregiver archetype 127
Cave (guided imagery) initiatives 106–10

Changing Points of View initiatives 65–70, 92–6
Charyton, C. 16–17
clay 19–20, 60
Cognitive/Symbolic level 14
cognitive variable 13
Cohen, Barry 6
Cohen, Felice 5
collage initiatives.
    See Powerful and Powerless Collage initiative; Rhyne's Problem-Solving Collage initiative
compensatory play 15
concrete thinkers 25
copying, act of 160–1
creativity
    art and 167–71
    decrease in 171
    defined 8
    drawing without thinking 161–2
    education and 165–7
    as ETC variable 14
    exercises 160–3
    promotes discovery 170
    science and 165
creativity activation
    battle drawing 136
    body tracing 120
    box self 117
    bridges 157
    caves 110
    changing perspective 162
    changing points of view 70, 95
    collage initiatives 140, 143
    defined 171
    dyadic nonverbal communication 56
    environmental awareness 113
    expressions in movement and sound 32
    expressive drawings 51–2
    in Expressive Therapies Continuum 160
    family-of-origin sculpture 147
    guided imagery 100
    haptic/visual self symbol 64

how I see myself/how others see me 59
images of pain and healing 75
lifeline initiative 124–5
mandalas 79, 81
media properties 36–7
my role in life 129
as new way of thinking 159
personal masks 133
scribble drawing 27
survival on an island 153
visual breathing 43
word initiative 91
Creator archetype 127

data management 160
design, elements of 141
Destroyer archetype 127
developmental art group 11
divergent thinking 32
Dondis, D. 46
drawing without thinking 161–2
dual mandalas 82
Dwelling (guided imagery) initiatives 101–5
Dyadic Nonverbal Communication initiative 53–6

ecstasy 163
education and creativity 165–7
Ego archetypes 126–7
Emotions
  compartmentalizing 17
  drawings representing 49–50
  identifying 72
  impacting breathing 44
  integrating contrasting 71
  survival function of 14
  visual language and 46, 48
Environmental Awareness initiative 111–14
environmental boundaries 9
Explorer archetype 127
Expressions in Movement and Sound initiative 29–33, 173
Expressions of Healing; Embracing the Process of Grief (Graves) 121
Expressive Drawings: Mind States-Mood States initiative 46–52
expressive therapies, interrelationship among 6
Expressive Therapies Continuum (ETC)
  creativity activation in 160
  developmental structure of 13
  foundations of 13–16
  Graphic Development and 20
  integration and continuum of concepts 20–1
  Play Development and 20
  resonance 164
  variables 13–14
Expressive Therapies Summit 6
eye (symbol) 78

Family-of-Origin Sculpture initiative 145–7
fear 14
Fincher, Suzanne 76
finger paints 18
flow, defined 163
fluid materials 18, 25
free association 91

Gestalt art therapy 18, 46
glad (mood state) 50
graphic development 15–16, 20, 173
Graves, Sandra 121
grief 121
groups 166
group work 27, 148–9
guided imagery
  adaptation of 110
  encouraging visuals 153
  memory recollection and 162
  symbolic choices 102–4, 107
  use of 95–6
guided imagery initiatives
  adaptation of 174
  cave 106–10
  dwelling 101–5
  source 97–100, 105
Gypsy of the soul 127

happiness 14, 72
Haptic/Visual Self Symbol initiative 60–4
Hero archetype 127
High Complexity Unstructured Resistive (HCUR) 32
higher-functioning residents 11
Hissom Memorial Center 2–3
Howard, Margaret 2, 5
How I See Myself/How Others See Me initiative 57–9
Huang, T. L. 16–17

idea generation 59, 64 *See also* creativity activation
illumination 52, 64, 70
images, power of 100
Images of Pain and Healing initiative 71–5
imagination 43, 100, 110, 127, 165
inner conflicts 134
Innocent archetype 126–7
Institute of Expressive Therapies 6
intuitive voice 160
isomorphism 17

Jones, Don 5
Jung, Carl 126
Jungian archetypes 126

Kim, Kyung Hee 171
Kinesthetic/Sensory level 14, 23
kinesthetic variable 13
Kotler, S. 163

Landgarten, Helen 5
Leland, Henry 4
Levick, Myra 5
Lifeline initiative 121–5
linear thinking 124–5
liquidating play 15
loss 121
Lover archetype 127
Lowenfeld, Viktor 6, 14, 15
Lusebrink, Vija 6
Lyons, J. 48

mad (mood state) 49
Magician archetype 128
Malchiodi, Cathy 21
Mandala, the Great Round initiative
 adaptation 81–5
 creativity activation 79, 81
 directives 77
 examples 77, 79, 83–5
 materials 77
 rationale 77–8
 "single eye" symbol 78
 symbolism 78
 therapeutic transition 78, 80–1
 visual word 82
 word-insertion mandala 86
mandalas
 defined 76
 dual 82

 example of 83–5
 visual word 82
 word-insertion 86
Mandala Symbolism (Jung) 76
Martínez Ayala, Gloria 76
martyrdom 127
Media Dimension Variables (MDV)
 art behavior reinforcement group 10–11
 concept of 4, 5, 8, *21*
 physical properties of 10
 rating scale 36
 sorting task 10–11
 structure of 9
 task complexity of 9
media/materials
 boundary determined 19
 clay 19–20, 60
 to create action 18, 162–3
 defined 19
 evaluating response to 17–18
 fluid 18, 25
 manipulating 9
 as metaphors 18
 mixed media 35
 paints 35, 65
 papers 34–5
 physical properties of 9–10
 quantity determined 19
 restrictive materials 10
Media Properties and Range of Materials initiative 34–7, 173
memory recollection 162
mental processes, described 17
Merryman, A. 171
mindfulness 39, 111
mindset 159–60
movement exercises 28
Mueller, Elsie 5
My Role in Life initiative 128–9

natural clay stoneware 19–20
naturalism 16
Naumburg, Margaret 2
nonverbal communication 53, 56
 See also dyadic nonverbal communication initiative

Orphan archetype 127

paint, use of 65
paintings, as metaphor 65

Parrish, Robert 1
Parsons State Hospital 4
pathological behaviors 111
Perceptual/Affective level 14
perceptual variable 13
personal fantasy 112
personal unconscious 20
Persona Masks initiative 130–3
perspective 162
Piaget, Jean 14
Piaget's developmental sequences 14
Play Development 20
Ploger, Ben 5
polarities 46
Powerful and Powerless Collage initiative 137–40
powerlessness 137
practice play 14, 15
preschematic stage 15
prestructured object, use of 115
problem solving
   ambiguity and 75
   by changing perspectives 92–3
   collage initiatives 137–44, 168–9
   dissecting the issue 142
"process as the self" 18
psychiatric group 11
psychodynamically oriented art therapy 4

realism 16
Realistic Stage 16
Rebel archetype 127
reflective distance 122
regression 15, 25, 32
resiliency 14, 25, 71
resolution 164–5
resonance 16, 17, 164–5
restrictive materials 59
retreating response 56
Rhyne, Janie 18, 46
Rhyne's Problem-Solving Collage initiative 141–4
Robinson, Ken 170–1
role playing 145, 147
Ronnberg, Ami 98
Ruler archetype 128

sadness 14, 48–9
Sage archetype 128
scared (mood state) 50
Scheere, M. 48

schema, described 15
schematic ranges of development 15–16
science, technology, engineering, and math (STEM) education 172
Science, Technology, Engineering, Art, and Mathematics (S.T.E.A.M.) education 172–4
science and creativity 165
Scribble Chase Mural initiative 24–8, 173
scribble drawing 15, 24
Seeker archetype 127
self, the
   conflicting sides of 133
   different personas of 115
   exploration of 164–5
   integration of 109–10
   prestructured object representing 115
   "process as the self" 18
   roles of family on 145
   through creativity 164–5
Self archetypes 128
self-awareness 118
self-empowerment 137
self-image 118
self-perception 57, 115–17
sensorimotor play 14, 15
sensorimotor stage of cognitive development 23
sensory operant stimulation [SOS] movement 3
sensory variable 13
shadow self 130
Siegel, Dan 111
Siegel, David 17, 21
"single eye" symbol 78
Socialization and Self-Image group 11
sorting task 10–11
Soul archetypes 127
sound, expressions in 173
"Special Child's View, A" art show 11
state of mind 48
STEAM education 172–4
Stites, Raymond 4
structured tasks 10–11
structure properties of MDV 9
Survival on an Island initiative 148–53, 166–7
symbolic variable 13
symbolism
   bridges as 154

environmental 112
in guided imagery 102–4, 107
Jungian perspective on 20
of mandalas 78
"single eye" as 78

tactile experience 145
task complexity of MDV 9
task directions 9
team-building 148–9, 166
therapeutic transition
  Battle Drawing initiative 135
  Body Tracing initiative 120
  Box Self (Inner/Outer Self) initiative 117
  Bridge initiative 155, 157
  The Cave (guided imagery) initiative 109–10
  Changing Points of View 1 initiative 69–70
  Changing Points of View 2 initiative 95
  The Dwelling (guided imagery) initiative 105
  Dyadic Nonverbal Communication initiative 55–6
  Environmental Awareness initiative 113
  Expressions in Movement and Sound initiative 31–2
  Expressive Drawings: Mind States-Mood States initiative 51
  Family-of-Origin sculpture initiative 146
  Haptic/Visual Self Symbol initiative 62–3, 64
  How I See Myself/How Others See Me initiative 59
  Images of Pain and Healing initiative 75
  Lifeline initiative 124
  Mandala, the Great Round initiative 78, 80–1
  My Role in Life initiative 129
  Persona Masks initiative 132–3
  Powerful and Powerless Collage initiative 139
  Scribble Chase Mural initiative 26–7
  The Source (guided imagery) initiative 100
  Survival on an Island initiative 153
  Visual Breathing initiative 43
  Word initiative, 91
thinking patterns 167
tolerance for ambiguity 51–2, 59, 70
Torrance Tests of Creative Thinking (TTCT) 171
truth seeker 128

Ulman, Elinor 3, 5
University of Louisville 5–6
unstructured projects 10

Visual Breathing initiative 38–44,
visual constructs 173
visual language 25, 48
visual word mandala 82
voice, intuitive 160

watercolor markers 18
White, Roger 5
Winnicott, D. W. 171
wise man 128
Word initiative, The 90, 168–9
word-insertion mandala 86

zone hackers 159–60